A WOMAN'S INITIATION

A WOMAN'S INITIATION

Women's Experiences with Breast Cancer
and How It Transformed Their Lives

Diana Murphy, MA, MFT

A Woman's Initiation: *Women's Experiences With Breast Cancer and How It Transformed Their Lives*
By Diana Murphy MA, MFT

Published by:
Synchronicity Books
18340 Sonoma Highway
Sonoma, California 95476
(707) 939-9212

Publisher's Cataloging-in-Publication
(Provided by Quality Books, Inc.)

Murphy, Diana, 1951-
  A woman's initiation : women's experiences with breast cancer and how it transformed their lives / Diana Murphy.
    p. cm.
    LCCN 2006902987
    ISBN 0-9779556-0-5

  1. Breast--Cancer--Patients--United States--Biography. 2. Breast--Cancer--Psychological aspects.
  I. Title.

RC280.B8M86 2006   362.196'99449'00922
                        QBI06-600136

In loving memory

of Patricia Kunz

ACKNOWLEDGEMENTS

I would like to thank Simon, Kate and Cierra for creating a beautiful book in spite of me; Kathlene Carney for getting the word out; Alice Acheson for sharing her wisdom and experience; Lowry McFerrin and Linda Watanabe McFerrin for their endless support and encouragement; Leslie Ghirla, Uma Macfarlane, Lisa Powers, Lori Ross and Mary Webber for arranging interviews for me. Most of all I want to thank everyone who shared their breast cancer experiences with me. And I want to thank my neighbor, Roney Wiseman, for teaching me how to use a computer and for providing ongoing tech support.

CONTENTS

INTRODUCTION

Our culture is sadly devoid of ritual, particularly rite-of-passage ritual. Certainly we have our confirmations and bar mitzvahs. But what have we to compare with a young man's journey into the woods, without food or a weapon to defend himself, risking death at the capricious hand of nature, to wait for a dream to come, to transform him. In the woods, in a sense, he does die. His old self dies and his new self is born. When he returns to the village he will have a new name and a new self. Villagers won't recognize him at first, and need to make his acquaintance anew.

One of the few things we have, powerful enough to transform our naysayer selves is life-threatening illness. The high-powered executive, invincible one minute, doubled over with excruciating chest pains the next. He lies in his hospital bed, his bare buttocks hanging out of his gown, his needs at the mercy of a nurse's aide, with her GED, who calls him "honey." He too has died, but for the time being, rebirth eludes him.

The woman who was raised to believe that only motherhood truly fulfills a woman, delayed marriage in favor of career, then motherhood until she and her husband were financially ready. She's diagnosed with breast cancer. Chemotherapy will be required. Chemo will leave her sterile. Her old self has also died.

In this disassociated state many try frantically to reconstruct what was, to get on with life as if nothing happened. Others slip into despair, as yet another blow has leveled their already wretched lives.

Some allow death, not without considerable resistance initially, allowing the experience to pierce and burn through them, stripping away that which they should have been, tried to be, pretended to be, to finally allow their true selves to emerge.

Life-threatening illness leads to a particularly poignant initiation when a person is between 40 and 55, primed for mid-life transition.

Mid-life tends to be precipitated by the catastrophic: the perfect marriage that endured twenty years of life's challenges suddenly falls apart because the couple has grown in different directions; the woman who invested her life in motherhood is left in an empty nest; the loyal employee of thirty years receives a generous severance package and a farewell handshake. As in life-threatening illness, the vehicle through which these people have defined their lives has been ripped from them. They flounder, without a purpose or an identity.

Life-threatening illness throws an extra punch into the mid-life experience, the direct experience of mortality. Whether one is in reality "healthy as a horse," with a good fifty years ahead, or gravely ill with metastatic cancer, hoping for five more, the message is the same: Life is a terminal illness and death is the ultimate outcome. Life-threatening illness hammers the point home.

Breast cancer is a female-specific mid-life initiation. It threatens all that traditionally defines a woman: fertility and motherhood, the vixen sexuality and maidenly beauty of youth. Even a mild run-in with breast cancer leaves psychic scars. One woman who had a lumpectomy and radiation was so devastated by the surgical deformity and radiation scarring of her breast, she resolved to keep her body hidden away and never take another lover.

Breast cancer is the great equalizer. Breastless, and bald, women are stripped of the board-room blue suit, surgical scrubs, nun's habit, and G-string and pasties. What remains is the primal feminine, which is both universal and unique. In support groups, women from divergent walks of life, who would never meet under ordinary circumstances, are thrown together to painfully and lovingly acknowledge their sameness and help each other to facilitate healing and growth that lead to a more genuine sense of self, unrelated to ornamentation or plumbing.

When a woman is diagnosed with breast cancer she enters those same woods, alone, without a weapon to defend herself. Her body will be dissected by scalpels, burned by radiation and mutilated by deadly chemicals. If she can reach into the depths of herself to find the courage and faith to withstand the ordeal and wait for the dream to come to transform her, breast cancer will become a woman's initiation.

I

WORK IS WHERE THE HEART IS

NAOMI

WHEN THE STUDENT IS READY
THE TEACHER ARRIVES

"I did it all right. I never should have gotten cancer," Naomi insisted. "I ate an organic vegetarian diet, exercised, never smoked, rarely drank. I even had my first child a few months before I turned 30, and I breast-fed."

Naomi is unquestionably a no-nonsense woman, from her easy-to-care-for, cropped hair, to her sensible shoes. With a doctorate in biochemistry, she views life as a series of solvable equations. Breast cancer skewed the picture.

Naomi grew up in New Jersey, "the hotbed of cancer." "My father died of lung cancer, my mother colon cancer, and a sister, leukemia. The only relative who got breast cancer was my aunt. It was the early seventies and all they did were radical mastectomies. She lost both breasts, was horribly scarred. The worst thing, though, was the lymphedema. Her arms looked like she had elephantiasis. And she was only 39. Cancer really scared me.

"I remember the pesticide trucks coming through every afternoon and spraying the neighborhood. It's a wonder everyone in New Jersey doesn't get cancer. I got the hell out as soon as I could."

A superior student, Naomi's intellect was her ticket out. She earned a full undergraduate scholarship. She chose the University of California, Berkeley, as far away from New Jersey as she could get.

She went from undergraduate to graduate school, and earned her doctorate in biochemistry. In graduate school she met Richard, a studious, unemotional man. They married shortly after graduation and settled into a quiet, predictable life together.

Their marriage, their lives and their careers were unfolding according to plan. Then breast cancer came along, and burst open their safe, predictable world.

"It's funny, in retrospect," Naomi recalls, "how I tried to intellectualize my way through cancer. I was 44 when I went in for my biannual mammogram. The film showed some irregularity, so the doctor had me come back for more detailed pictures. I was premenopausal and had very fibrous breasts. I assumed that it was nothing."

She had a sonogram and a needle biopsy that revealed a very small, 2 mm, invasive tumor, and a larger, 1 cm, ductile carcinoma in situ (DCIS).

"I cried a little when I got my results," Naomi remembers. "Then my scientific mind took over, and I went into action. I called my doctor friends and collected referrals to surgeons. Then I interviewed them and found someone I liked. The surgery date was set for a week later. I spent that week becoming an expert on breast cancer. I learned that I would be having a lumpectomy, followed by radiation. I felt comfortable, because I knew what to expect; or so I thought.

"While I was staying in control at first, my calm, rational husband was anything but. I had never seen Richard cry; not in movies like *Philadelphia*, where the whole audience is crying; not when his father died the year before.

"The day I got my diagnosis I didn't call him at work. I didn't want to bother him. I waited until he got home to tell him. I expected him, as usual, to be my rock. Instead, he burst into tears. I remember thinking, 'Great, now I'll have to be the strong one for both of us.'"

Naomi went into surgery calm and in control. Then she got her results. Although the invasive tumor was small, there was nodal involvement. This meant chemotherapy.

"Chemo terrified me. I saw my parents and my sister go through it: retchingly ill, too weak to move, and each of them died anyway. People told me that chemo was much better than it used to be in the seventies and eighties. I didn't believe it, and I didn't want any part of it."

Naomi's surgeon referred her to a top oncologist, who recommended a six-treatment chemotherapy regime. She sought two second opinions. Both oncologists made exactly the same recommendation.

"I spent a month trying to find someone to agree with me, that I didn't need it, or at least recommend fewer treatments. I just wanted to have acupuncture. Nobody was going for that.

"Poor Richard was so afraid that I was going to die if I didn't have it. He and the kids were trying to coerce me, right along with the doctors. I felt like I got dragged to chemo, kicking and screaming, by the people who love me the most."

Naomi's chemotherapy experience was a particularly bad one. The chemo made her sick. The anti-nausea drugs made her sicker. She had treatment every three weeks and spent ten days after each one in bed, too weak to function.

"After the third treatment I was lying in bed one night and this feeling rushed over me. It … it was like a failure to thrive. I could no longer tolerate being in my body, and really thought that one more treatment would kill me.

"I refused to continue treatment. I was too weak to speak for myself. Even though he disagreed with me, and was worried sick that if I didn't complete the regime I'd die, Richard spoke for me. The doctor said I had to finish the treatment. She changed the drugs and referred me to an acupuncturist who specializes in breast cancer.

"I made it through the last three treatments and started to recover quickly. The tide had finally turned. What I didn't realize at the time was that meeting Grace, the acupuncturist, was going to change my life.

"After enduring chemo, I had had it with the medical profession. Working with Grace was so different. To her, medicine was an art, not a science. As a scientist myself I'm leery of anything that seems to be the least bit 'airy-fairy New Age.' But this wasn't. I felt comfortable with acupuncture as a valid healing technique, and Grace, as a healer, from the get-go.

"Grace doesn't rely on laboratory tests. She studied my pulse, examined my tongue, my hands, my eyes. Most of all she asked me a lot of questions about me — not my disease, me. And, she really listened to my answers. With the help of acupuncture I recovered quickly and was able to get back to my healthy lifestyle."

Naomi's life seemed to get back to normal. She'd put the whole experience of cancer behind her, as if it had never happened. Then she went in for her next mammogram.

There was a cloudy spot on the film, on her other breast. A needle biopsy revealed DCIS.

"This time I completely lost it. I cried. I screamed. Poor Richard, who had gone with me, had never in our almost twenty years of marriage, seen me out of control. He had no idea what to do.

"I had succumbed to chemo, against my will. I'd suffered, but I hadn't quit. I went to acupuncture. I got my health and my healthy lifestyle back. How the hell could I have gotten cancer again?

"My surgeon said that the DCIS had probably been there all along. Before chemo I wasn't menopausal, and my breasts were denser. The earlier mammogram had missed it. Since DCIS doesn't respond to chemo, it was still there.

"No dice. I wasn't buying a rational, logical answer. Logic and reason had failed me. Control had failed me. Everything I had counted on to keep my life running smoothly, on track, had failed me. I was mad as hell about it."

Naomi had a second surgery that easily removed the DCIS. But Naomi plunged into a severe depression. Richard tried to be there, but she was inconsolable. Finally, she decided to go to therapy.

"I had never considered therapy before," she recalls. "I'd gone to one breast cancer support group. It was too sad. The women were all worse than I was. At that point, I was just trying to slide through as quietly, and unconsciously, as possible. Now, I had no choice. I really had to look at what was going on.

"A friend referred me to a therapist who specializes in working with breast cancer survivors. Emily, the therapist, assured me that nothing that I was going through was abnormal. I had a perfect right to be angry. Our task together was to get below the anger and see what was causing it — what the experience with breast cancer had to teach me."

In therapy, Naomi had to journey back to the people and place she had long left behind, and tried to pretend never existed at all, her family in New Jersey.

Naomi was the oldest of three children. Both of her parents were alcoholic and abusive, to each other and their children. Many nights Naomi would hole up in her room, curled up in bed, hugging her younger sisters. Downstairs there was a symphony of frenzied, pitched screams and breaking glass.

As is typical for children of alcoholics, Naomi constructed an illusion of protection, by always being very much in control. As an intelligent child and superior student by nature, she gravitated towards math and science, where there was always a formula and a right answer.

Her full scholarship to UC Berkeley was her ticket out of New Jersey, and her family life, once and for all. She created a safe, predictable lifestyle for herself that involved a lot of studying and healthy living (atypical of a college student). At last, she felt safe.

In the doctoral program she met Richard, a quiet, reserved man, who was 180 degrees from her violent, raging father. They were each other's first love interest (probably more appropriately, each other's first security and compatibility interest). They married shortly after graduate school.

Unlike Naomi, Richard had grown up in a cold, reserved family, where members barely acknowledged each other's presence. A woman like Naomi, who kept herself feeling safe with a controlled, orderly life, offered a level of intimacy he could safely tolerate. Each had met their match.

When breast cancer threatened Naomi's life, a radical shift took place in Richard. Below the surface of respect and compatibility, a genuine love had grown. When the prospect of losing Naomi arose, an emotional levee broke in Richard.

Naomi, on the other hand, had needed the strong fortress of control to face the agony of cancer treatment. Only when her illusion of control failed her did her own emotional levee break.

"Richard and I started fighting all the time. We'd always been one of those couples who never fought. Now, we were fighting about nothing.

"I always carefully wash the coffeepot after I use it, then put it back on the coffee maker. One Sunday morning Richard put it back without washing it. I flew into a rage, calling him lazy, slovenly and insensitive. He called me a controlling, anal-retentive bitch. We went on and on until he slammed the door and left. Later, we talked about it and decided that we should see a couple's therapist, before whatever was going on tore our marriage apart.

"So, here I was in individual therapy and couple's therapy. Me, the one who never wanted to look at what was going on, got dragged there, kicking and screaming, by cancer. All of it helped. But, what helped most was acupuncture; not exactly acupuncture, but Grace.

"Grace and I would have these long talks when I went in for treatment. She's been a Buddhist for over twenty years. She'd say things like, 'The root of all suffering is attachment.' I was going through hell, because I'd been attached to control for so long. When I finally had to accept that I couldn't control my life, I fell apart. Falling apart was the beginning of coming together in a more authentic whole.

"A few years ago I wouldn't have listened to a word of it. Sometimes the curmudgeon in me still refuses to go there. But I needed to believe in something, and I trusted Grace. When I didn't understand something she would say, 'When the student's ready, the teacher arrives.' This I really didn't understand. I wanted to understand, now. The last thing I wanted to do was to wait patiently for understanding to come. Grace would just smile."

Not having been given a choice in the matter, Naomi waited. She waited and she worked hard in her own therapy, and in couple's work with Richard. They learned that much of that which attracted them to each other was safety. Meanwhile, they had grown to love each other. When cancer forced each of them to change and grow as individuals, what felt "safe" in their marriage before, felt constricting, even suffocating, now. With their therapist's help, they nurtured their relationship, and allowed it to grow and change, too.

Naomi had to face one more life transition. Fortunately, this one made its presence known fairly gently, seemingly naturally. She was working in the lab one afternoon, when a thought quietly entered her consciousness.

"I knew that I didn't want to do this work anymore. There wasn't anything wrong with the job. I worked for an ethical company that does medical research. It's work I can feel proud of. But it had come to feel too limiting, like I'd outgrown it. I went into science because it was full of certainty, provability that let me feel secure. Working in the lab, there is a minimal amount of human interaction. It's not like you have to deal with organizational politics; you just close the door and do your job. Now, I wanted human interaction. I wanted to use my scientific knowledge to work directly with people. I wanted to be a healer."

That evening she and Richard discussed it. Since she had a long-term positive relationship with her employer, she would probably be able to cut down her hours to part-time. They might even be willing to reimburse her for some of her education. Since she had a doctorate in science she would be able to waive some of the required courses, and start with the hands-on classes and apprenticing. Richard supported her 100%. If he wanted to make a career change down the line she promised to support him.

Then she picked up the phone and made a call. "The student is ready, but the teacher has always been there. I want to apprentice with you."

Grace wasn't surprised.

STEPHANIE

TURNING HER BACK ON SUCCESS

"Cancer is inconvenient," Stephanie laughed.

She was 45 at the time of her diagnosis. Her ugly, two-year divorce was final. A few months earlier she had been promoted: the first woman at the bank to make senior vice president.

Stephanie is a strikingly attractive woman: slim, gym-fit, with perfectly coifed honey-blond hair and piercing green eyes. Her suit is Chanel, her shoes Jimmy Choo, her handbag real Prada. Nothing in her appearance suggests a girl who came up the hard way.

The oldest of two children, she was nine when her parents divorced, and her mother fell apart. She had to grow up quickly, to raise herself and her younger sister. She started working at 16. At 18 she got a job as a bank teller. In an era of MBAs and management training, she rose through the ranks to become the first female senior vice president. Now her very foundation felt threatened.

She had gone for her yearly OB-GYN examination. The doctor felt a lump. "I can't possibly have cancer," she vividly remembers thinking. "I'm too new at the job, too easy to replace. I'm single. I can't lose a breast. I thought about how cancer would impact my career, my marriageability. It never occurred to me that it could cost me my life."

Her diagnosis was ductile carcinoma in situ (DCIS). At that point in time, it was a hotly debated issue in cancer circles, whether

DCIS was in fact cancer or a precancerous condition.

In her mind, this let Stephanie off the hook. She didn't have to have cancer. She only had a precancerous condition. She would have it taken care of quickly and quietly. She'd get right back to business as usual, and no one would be the wiser.

"Breast conservation was my primary concern," she said. "The deeper medical ramifications just seemed to slide by me." She had three lumpectomies, each six months apart. It took three surgeries to get clear margins.

"Each time I'd tell my staff that I was having oral surgery, take off Wednesday through Friday, and come back to work on Monday. They must have thought I had the worst teeth in town."

She went through each surgery alone, and told no one. "I'd take a cab to and from the hospital, make sure I had enough food, pain pills and DVDs to get through, until I was good enough to go back to work."

After the third surgery the doctor recommended radiation and tamoxafin. She declined radiation because it would be too time-consuming, and she feared that it would shrivel up the breast. She was willing to go on tamoxafin.

"After the last surgery I just wanted to put all of this 'cancer stuff' behind me and get back to my life. But tamoxafin put me in menopause. It wasn't just hot flashes and night sweats, it was my looks. My skin was drying up and wrinkling like an old prune. My vagina was as dry as wood. I had no desire and sex hurt like hell. I wondered whether life without estrogen was worth living.

"I went from oncologist to oncologist, until I found one who was liberal enough to put me on HRT. His reasoning was that the tamoxafin was blocking the estrogen to my breasts; there was no reason the rest of me needed to suffer."

HRT not withstanding, she only lasted a year on tamoxafin. "I still felt and looked menopausal. I was afraid I was losing my femininity, and I couldn't take it. I also got very depressed. I cried all the time, had trouble sleeping, trouble getting up in the morning."

Her primary care doctor put her on antidepressants and recommended psychotherapy. "At that point," she said, "I didn't want to understand it. I just wanted to fix it. I was single, menopausal and miserable. I just wanted to feel good enough to throw myself back into my work." She went on antidepressants, and that's exactly what she did.

A year later, she met Jack while working out at the gym. Jack was a fireman, who was writing his first novel.

"I found Jack attractive, and thought he was a great guy. But, I knew I could never get serious about him. He just wasn't my type. I only dated upscale businessmen. I still figured that Jack and I could be friends."

They'd go out for coffee or a glass of wine after their workouts. Both avid runners, they'd go for their Saturday long runs together and then go out for breakfast.

"We'd go for a run and have these great talks. Jack was a widower. He told me that his first wife had died of breast cancer. He had taken care of her through it all and it had been pretty hard on him. I guess, unconsciously, I knew there was more to it than friendship, because I made sure not to tell him about my brush with cancer."

After a year or so as "friends," their relationship did develop into more. "It was the most intimate, honest relationship I've ever had with a man. It was wonderful and scary at the same time. Until then I hadn't given cancer recurrence a second thought. Now, I really had something to lose."

When Stephanie went for her five-year clinical breast exam, she said, "I had a really bad feeling. Maybe it was just superstition on my part. Or maybe, for the first time in my life, I really felt like I had something to live for."

The doctor felt something. She ordered a mammogram, then a needle biopsy. The cancer had recurred.

"I was devastated," she said, "confused, angry, scared. You name it, I felt it, and all at once. I couldn't tell Jack. On one hand, I was afraid he'd leave. On the other, I was afraid he'd stay and I'd die. I just couldn't do that to him. I just wanted to run away from all of it."

It took her three weeks to tell him. They were lying in bed on a Sunday morning. She turned towards him, her voice shaking. "Honey, there's… there's something I have to tell you. I… I have br… br…

breast cancer."

They held each other, both crying, for the longest time. Then, Jack said, "We'll get through this together." Then they both cried some more.

The doctors offered Stephanie another lumpectomy or a mastectomy with reconstruction. "I couldn't see them chipping away at it any longer. Since I would have reconstruction at the same time I opted for the mastectomy."

The date was set. Jack stayed with Stephanie the night before, and drove her to the hospital. He stayed with her through the pre-op, holding her hand as they wheeled the gurney down the hall. Finally, they let go of each other's hands, and she was wheeled through the doors of the operating room.

In the surgery, the doctors found nodal involvement, which raised the cancer to level II and meant that chemotherapy would be required. "I was terrified at the thought of having chemo," she said. "All those toxic chemicals floating around in my body, losing my hair. And it was every bit as horrible as I'd expected.

"Some days I felt so sick I thought I'd just curl up on the couch and stay there all day. And that's exactly what I'd do. My golden retriever, Maggie, would curl up next to me and the two of us would just lie there for hours. One night the vomiting was particularly bad. I just lay on the bathroom floor waiting for the next round. Maggie woke up and heard me. She came into the bathroom and quietly lay down next to me.

"Chemo strips you of everything. I'd planned to take three weeks off work, have the mastectomy and get back to business as usual. I ended up taking a one-year leave of absence. I went from working sixty to eighty hours a week, to lying on the couch too ill to move for hours on end. I'd defined myself by work since I was 16. Now, I was 50 and I no longer knew who I was, or who I'd be when this thing was over (or if I'd be here when it was over).

Stephanie went back to work three months after chemo ended. She felt ready, even looked forward to it. She planned to approach work differently, to delegate authority, and not carry all the weight herself. "My staff did a stellar job without me. They clearly don't need my micro-managing, and I don't need it anymore either."

Despite her best efforts, the return to work wasn't easy. "I used to be so hyper and just threw myself into work. I can't do that anymore. I spent so many hours just being by myself when I was sick, I got used to it. I need time for me in my life. Although my approach to work is more relaxed, more laissez-faire, I honestly find that I just don't want to be there."

Stephanie felt like she was having some sort of existential crisis. She had expected to go from being totally work-focused to being more relaxed at work, not wanting to dump the job altogether. She turned to therapy, and with the kind of energy she had previously devoted to her job, she sought to explore and solve the dilemma.

"What I discovered surprised me," she said. "When I started working at 16, it wasn't because I wanted to. My love was art. I'd won a couple of awards in school, and my teacher thought I could win a full scholarship to art school. But when my parents divorced, my mother got seriously depressed and pretty much stayed in bed all day. My dad paid alimony and child support, but it wasn't enough. I'd find bills unopened, and when I opened them we were ninety days past due, and they were going to cut off our electricity, and things like that. At first, I'd call my dad and he'd take care of it. Eventually, I didn't want to bother him, so I started paying the bills myself, from my part-time job at the café. I started working more and more hours, and in the summer I worked full-time, plus overtime.

"Art school just wasn't going to happen for me. When I graduated from high school I got a job as a teller. What I wanted wasn't important. I had responsibilities now. I just rolled up my sleeves and went to work. I worked hard and got promoted. I helped put my sister through college. My mother never really got better. Eventually, I had to put her in a board-and-care home.

"Now I'm 50. I've survived cancer. I've met the man I want to share my life with. I don't know if I have a long time to live, or a short time. All I know is that it's my turn now."

Stephanie and Jack will be getting married soon. They went to a financial planner to assess their fiscal situation. Jack will be fully vested and able to retire from the fire department in two years, so he can concentrate on his writing. It looks as if Stephanie will also be able to retire then, and give her art a real shot.

"We want to travel too," she said. "There are so many places I've never been. We plan to get to as many as possible.

"You know, breast cancer was really awful. I'm glad it's a thing of the past and hope that's where it stays. But it changed my life in so many good ways — things I probably would have never changed without it. It sounds funny to say, but in a way, cancer is the best thing that ever happened to me."

II

IT'S ALL IN THE FAMILY

CHRIS

WE'RE AN INTENTIONAL FAMILY

Chris is a tall, lanky, athletic woman with sandy blond hair and a perpetual tan. Even the sprigs of grey in her hair and crinkles around her eyes and mouth barely hint at her age, or how much she's been through in her 55 years.

Chris lives on a ranch in the mountains of Southern California with her life partner, Liz, one of their four adopted children, and numerous dogs, cats and farm animals.

"I always wanted to be a doctor, but I ran into a streak of ill health in college, a benign brain tumor and scarlet fever, that kept delaying me. I settled for a PhD in biology and became a college professor."

During the nineties, the college where Chris teaches experienced what appeared to be a cancer epidemic. "Eleven people in the administration building were stricken with some form of cancer, suggesting some serious environmental toxins in that building."

Back in the biology building, Chris's office-mate and good friend Marilyn had metastatic breast cancer. Two months after Marilyn died, Chris found a lump in her own right breast.

"In spite of the cancer epidemic at school I wasn't worried. My mother had five breast tumors removed, all benign. I lived a healthy lifestyle — never smoked or did drugs, rarely drank, ate healthy and exercised." Chris wasn't worried, but for her partner Liz and her sister Kathy it was another story. They were both sick with worry. "When I went in for my needle biopsy they offered me a Valium. I turned it down. I only wanted a local anesthetic so I could be fully present. Liz and Kathy fought over the Valium," she laughs. "Liz won and I had to drive her home."

When she got the results it was quite another story. She had an aggressive, fast-growing tumor. Kathy, whose husband Mack was in treatment for non-Hodgkin's lymphoma, encouraged Chris to meet with the pathologist and find out as much as she could about the cancer.

"The pathologist was happy to meet with me. I guess he spends most of his time in the basement of the hospital — rarely, if ever, seeing patients. He showed me my tumor under magnification. We decided jointly where we'd send it and what we'd have it tested for. It turned out to be stage III, Her-2 positive. The prognosis, according to all the literature I read, was poor."

Chris scheduled her mastectomy and her family began to make their plans.

"My oldest daughter, June, was pregnant. She asked her doctor to induce labor so that the baby would be born before my surgery and I could be present in the delivery room. When the doctor questioned her, she told him that he wouldn't want to deal with her if her baby was being born without her mother in the room. June gave birth three days before my surgery. I was the first to hold my new grandson, Joshua.

"The night before surgery, Liz and I were going out to the movies when I got a call from my next-to-youngest, Carrie, who's a college student. She told me I had to come over right now. I said that we were going to a movie. She told me to go to a later show. She needed me to come over first.

"I assumed that there was something wrong with her. She'd been recovering from a sports injury. When I got to her apartment she just held me and cried. She kept saying, 'Mama, you can't die. Please don't die. You're all I've got.' I reminded her that she had her fiancé, Steve, her brother and sisters, Liz, her grandparents. But she kept saying that they weren't me. She didn't want to lose her mom. I was very touched and I cried too."

Chris had her surgery and was recuperating at the ranch. Before she started chemotherapy, Chris, Liz, and their only child still living at home, five-year-old Becky, packed their things and moved to an apartment near the medical center.

"We celebrated Becky's fifth birthday at the ranch. We had all of the neighbors and their kids over. There was a big cake and lots of ice cream. We gave the kids rides on our gentle pony, Scooter. Then we left it in the capable hands of our son, Jason, and moved to an apartment in town. I tried my best to hide my tears. I was afraid that I'd never see the ranch again.

"Chemotherapy scared the hell out of me; I have a genetic disease where my white blood cell count tends to go very low. I needed a lot of extra monitoring and special drugs, with unpredictable side effects, during chemo.

"Liz was working full-time, so I spent most of my days at home with Becky. We would play games. We wore elaborate costumes that she'd send Liz out to buy, and made stage props she created with the furniture. She'd dress me up and tell me what part to play. She taught me how to play. As a child I never played. I was a serious kid, an over-achiever. I wanted to make my parents proud of me. Deep down I thought there was something different or wrong with me. I was too young to understand what it meant to be gay. I just knew I needed to give my parents something else to be proud of. Little did I know how much I underestimated them or how supportive they'd be years later when I came out.

"At one point the chemo got so bad that Liz had to take the mattress off our bed and put it on the floor close to the bathroom. I only had enough strength left to crawl to the bathroom when I needed to puke."

Chris finished chemo and slowly began to recover. A year later in a CAT scan the doctor found a mass on one of her ovaries and didn't hesitate to recommend a full hysterectomy. Chris recalls, "After chemo, a hysterectomy was nothing."

After another recovery period, Chris was strong enough to move back to the ranch. Shortly after, she was ready to go back to teaching.

"It was really touching when I was sick that my students really came to the plate for me. They brought us food, ran errands. These kids reminded me of why I love teaching so much.

"I'm back teaching full-time now, but I'm to go part-time next year. My retirement will be fully vested then. If anything happens to me it will be there to take care of my kids.

"I'd pretty much been a workaholic all of my life. Cancer ground me to a halt. More important than that, it showed me how precious my family is. Liz, my kids, my parents, all gave me so much love and support. I couldn't have made it without them.

"I want to spend time on my ranch with my family. My dad died, God rest his soul, when I was recovering from my hysterectomy. I want my mom to come and live with us. She's part of the family, too. We're an intentional family, two middle-aged lesbians, four adopted, biracial kids, and lots of animals. We've made it work. It took cancer for me to realize that my family is the most important thing in my life.

"I'm five years in remission. I'd be a liar if I said that I didn't worry about the future. I liken cancer to a rattlesnake in my house. You can hear it, but you don't know where it is. I get a headache, I think brain tumor. My bones ache, I think bone cancer. But you can't live like that. It'll make you crazy. So most of the time I don't.

"Joyce, one of the breast cancer survivors from administration, had six years of remission. In those years she met a wonderful man. They got married and started building their dream house. Then the cancer recurred and she was diagnosed metastatic. She lived for three more years, saw her only daughter give birth, held her first grandchild.

"Joyce's story really scares me. She had a year more of remission than I do. But, it gives me hope, too. She lived nine years with breast cancer and she made them rich, wonderful years. That's what really matters most."

BILLIE SUE

CENTERFOLD TURNS BREAST CANCER ACTIVIST

To say that Billie Sue gets noticed when she enters a room is a huge understatement. Five feet, six inches of curves, poured into tight black capri pants and an equally tight, hot pink tee shirt with stiletto-heel sandals, big blond hair and long acrylic fingernails to match her pink tee — Billie Sue stands out in a crowd.

"I enjoy being a sexy woman. And I enjoy getting attention," she smiles. "But I've been happily married to the same man for twenty years, so it's just attention."

Billie Sue came from a family of large-breasted women. As a scrawny, flat-chested teenager, the boys ignored her. She continually pestered her mother, asking her when she was going to develop. "All in good time," her mother would tell her.

"Then," she recalls, "the summer I was 16 my boobs blossomed. When I went back to school the boys noticed. I got real popular, real quick."

As a young woman Billie Sue learned how to use her 40DD assets. She worked as a lingerie model, spent time as a cheerleader for a pro football team, and even posed once for a centerfold. Then she met Bob, a general contractor. They married, and she got her real estate license. She settled comfortably into a lifestyle of a wife, realtor, and eventually, mother.

As Billie Sue got older she learned that there was a price to pay for a voluptuous body. In her late 30s she developed back problems that didn't respond well to physical therapy. Her doctor suggested breast reduction.

"I was willing to have breast reduction to get relief from the pain I was in. My insurance would only pay for it if I was reduced to a B cup. A big part of my identity came from having big boobs. I only wanted my breast reduced to a C or D. So, I found a plastic surgeon and decided to pay for it myself."

The surgeon required that she have a mammogram before surgery. Billie Sue had never had a mammogram. She was only 39. There was no breast cancer in her family. Her doctor had never seen a reason to order one. In ordering one, the surgeon may very well have saved her life.

"The mammogram was really awful — my breasts being squeezed to death between those cold metal plates. I was relieved to get the whole thing over with. Then the next day I got a call to come in for a needle biopsy — no explanation, just come in at 11:30.

"The biopsy was even worse. It hurt so bad and I developed a hematoma. Little did I know the worst was still to come. I got a call the next day. The doctor told me I had breast cancer.

"I was hysterical. I'd only known one person who'd had breast cancer. Mrs. Jenkins. Both of my daughters had gone to the same schools and had many of the same teachers. Mrs. Jenkins was the first-grade teacher to both of them. She died six months after her diagnosis. We'd gone to her funeral two weeks before my diagnosis. I equated breast cancer with death.

"Even worse than trying to figure out how I was going to cope was figuring out how I was going to tell my daughters. When I told them, Tiffany, my 10-year-old, asked, 'Mommy, are you going to die, like Mrs. Jenkins?' I told her, 'Of course not,' and didn't believe a word I was saying."

Billie Sue had a lumpectomy and six weeks of radiation. The doctor told her she'd be ready to have a breast reduction six months later. He wanted to get another mammogram, just to be sure.

"I had the mammogram. Guess what showed up? Cancer: same

breast, same size (1 cm). It turns out that it was always there. The radiologist just missed it. I don't know how. I suppose I had cause for a malpractice suit. But I just wanted to take care of it, be done with cancer for good."

Billie Sue opted for a bilateral mastectomy with reconstruction. "The doctors said that they could save my nipples, but I just wanted to be rid of these things." She would discover that reconstruction is a lot more complicated when you've had radiation, because the skin loses its elasticity.

"I had these implants called expanders put in. At first you're completely flat, and then your boobs start to grow. Because my skin had lost elasticity it couldn't expand with the expander. I went to the mountains and the expander puffed up with the altitude. The implant burst and cut through my skin, leaking out all of this goop. I ended up having ten more surgeries to finally correct the problem." In the mastectomy the doctor found lymph node involvement. Billy Sue had to undergo six months of chemotherapy.

"Chemo was much worse than all the surgeries put together. I'd always been a really active person. Bob and the girls were used to my being up and at the gym by 5:00, back home with breakfast on the table before they got up. At first I tried to be up before they left for the day. After a few months I just tried to be out of bed by the time the girls got home from school. I succeeded about a third of the time.

"I learned that cancer brings out the best and the worst in people in your life. My close friends and family were wonderful. My 'man's man' husband was washing dishes, scrubbing toilets and attending our daughters' parent-teacher nights at school. My friends organized cooking and errand-running duties. Each day, fully cooked meals and any shopping I needed were left on the front porch. The next morning, empty food containers and new shopping lists were picked up.

"Strangers, on the other hand, could be awful. Right after I lost my hair I was in the restroom of a café. I'd washed my hands and was putting on my lipstick. A woman was standing behind me, watching me. When she went to turn on the faucet, she covered it with a paper towel. I felt just like a leper. I went out to my car and cried.

"The hardest thing was how cancer affected my relationship with my oldest daughter, Brittany. My youngest daughter, Tiffany, was only 10. She'd come home from school, climb in bed with me and we'd cuddle. But Brittany was 13. Her sexuality was just budding. She couldn't handle my losing my boobs and my hair. She'd barely come near me.

"I had always been a role model for my daughters. I was a wife and mother, a professional woman, but I was still sexy and glamorous. The mastectomy and chemo took my sexiness and glamour away. I hurt for both of us.

"I hated hurting my daughter, but it was as if she was holding up a mirror to me. I'd see this breastless, bald person with no eyebrows or eyelashes. I looked like a concentration camp victim. I wasn't a woman anymore. My identity had been my boobs and my looks. Without them I felt like I didn't exist anymore."

When Billie Sue had recovered sufficiently to get back to her life, she thought, 'Now what?' "I'd had it with lying around the house. I didn't want to go back to selling real estate. God had given me breast cancer for a reason. He had spared my life for a reason. What was it? What did He want me to do?

"I knew I wanted to give something back. So many people were there for me and I felt indebted. I wanted to help women going through what I'd been through. I thought about doing something to raise money for the Susan G. Komen Breast Cancer Foundation or the American Cancer Society. But I wanted to help who I wanted to help. I live in a rural area. We don't get the kind of attention from national foundations that cities do. I wanted to help women in my own county, so I started my own foundation."

Billie Sue needed a name for her foundation. She looked back on her breast cancer experience. Billie Sue's favorite flowers have always been red roses. After each chemo treatment, Bob would bring her a dozen red roses. Since it might be days before she was up to appreciating them, he always bought tight buds and put an aspirin in the water to keep them fresh for her.

"I'd lost my nipples in the mastectomy, but I was told that they can tattoo on phonies. I thought, hell, if I'm going to get my boobs tattooed I'm going for something more exciting than nipples. I had red roses. One thing led to another, and I named my foundation the Red Rose Foundation.

"The first cause that we championed was the Wellness Center, which had lost funding and was in jeopardy of closing. When I was going through treatment I went to support groups at the Wellness Center twice a week. It was the one place where I could safely take off my wig and let it all hang out. I couldn't allow this resource to be taken from other women in need."

The Red Rose Foundation sponsored a black-tie dinner and silent auction at the golf club. They raised $50,000 and kept the Wellness Center afloat.

Billie Sue and her foundation, staffed by volunteers, many of whom are Billie Sue's closest friends, went on to champion other causes. They raised funds for child care, house cleaning and meal-delivery services for women undergoing treatment in the county.

Billie Sue and her volunteers also go out and speak to women in the community, educating them about breast cancer, teaching them how to do self-exams, praising the value of mammograms. They speak at the PTA, a shopping mall, the Rotary Club, anywhere they can. Billie Sue is always quick to flip up her tee-shirt and show women that there is life after breast cancer. "I used to whip my top off at the slightest provocation. So God said, 'Okay, I'll give you breast cancer so when you whip your top off it's for a cause,'" Billie Sue laughs.

Billie Sue is approaching her five-year anniversary of remission. "Five years is a milestone, and I'm grateful. But I've known enough women who've had recurrences, even turned metastatic after five years. Breast cancer taught me that life is precious and short. It taught me the importance of the people in my life that I love.

"I've worked fifty to sixty hours a week at the foundation for the past two years. I'm proud of the foundation and what it's accomplished, and will accomplish in the future. But it's time for me to back off and let others carry the brunt.

"Working in real estate is demanding, and it took me away from my family. Then they lost me to breast cancer. The foundation turned into another way to deprive my family of my time.

"My girls are getting older. Brittany will be leaving for college in

the fall. We've never really bridged the impasse that breast cancer created. I hope it's not too late.

"Tiffany's in high school. She'll be gone soon enough and I want
to be a better mother to her than I could have been to Brittany. And
Bob was so wonderful through the whole thing. I don't think I'll ever
be able to show him how grateful I am.

"They say charity begins at home. My family's turn is long over-
due. That's where I want to direct my energy now."

GINA

AN ANGEL CAME TO VISIT ME

"I was 32 and I'd made a big decision. I was going to have breast-reduction surgery. I'd worn a 36DD since I was a teenager. I had the worst time buying clothes. I could never wear the cute little tops the other girls wore.

"I hated the male attention. I knew the boys were looking at my boobs, not me. When I got older, men were no better — well, except for my husband, Franklin, of course. He told me that if I wanted to have breast reduction, have it. He supported my decision. He loved me for me, not my boobs.

"A few days before I had surgery he took me shopping and bought me a beautiful strapless, emerald-green dress. I'd never worn anything like that in my life. He told me that after I recovered from surgery he'd take me dancing so I could show it off."

Gina is a petite, African-American woman with a broad smile, warm demeanor and plenty of spunk. In 1988, she endured a five-hour breast reduction surgery that took her breasts from a 36DD to a 36B. After the surgery, the breast tissue was sent to the lab. A week later Gina got a nasty surprise.

"The surgeon called me and told me I needed to come to his office. But, he didn't tell my why. I thought it was strange, because when I got there, Franklin was there. The surgeon had called my husband and told him that I had breast cancer, but he hadn't told me anything.

"The surgeon told both of us the good news. I had ductile carcinoma in situ, a type of breast cancer that is contained in the breast. Then he told us the bad news. I had several tumors throughout the breast and I would need to have a mastectomy. There were no other options.

"Franklin and I kept it together until we got out of the doctor's office. Then we went over to the park across the street and just held each other and cried. 'We'll get through this,' Franklin kept telling me."

Gina scheduled her surgery. She called her parents and members of her large extended family.

"My mom and my husband were great. But a lot of the other relatives acted really weird. The worst was a cousin who sat there in my hospital room doing her own breast self-exam while she was talking to me. I realized that most people, no matter how well intended, don't know what to say. They can end up saying or doing the worst possible things. I wanted to be around people who really knew what I was going through, so I joined a breast cancer support group through the American Cancer Society. The support group was such a big part of my recovery that afterwards I decided to train to become a volunteer counselor in their Reach Out to Recovery program.

"I'd go to meet with women in the hospital, or more often, in their homes. Nobody stays in the hospital very long anymore. I'd listen to their stories and tell them mine. I tried to answer their questions — anything from where to find a support group to who made the best wigs.

"It's sad. There's so much shame and secrecy about cancer, especially among black women. More white women are diagnosed with breast cancer, but black women die of it. I think the shame and secrecy are part of the reason. Some women hide it from everyone until it's progressed too far to do anything about it.

"I remember this one woman I telephoned. She told me that she was too embarrassed to have me come to her house and see her. She just wanted me to mail her the literature. I've always wondered what happened to her. Of course, I'll never know."

In the eighties, woman had to wait six months after a mastectomy before they could have reconstructive surgery. "Every day I had to stare at this hideous hole in my chest. It looked like a war wound. I'd stuff a falsie in my bra and half the time it would move and I'd end up with a shoulder pad. I'd go to the closet and look at my beautiful strapless dress and cry. I wondered if I'd ever wear it and have Franklin take me dancing."

Gina's recovery went well. She went for biannual clinical breast checkups and continued to volunteer for Reach Out to Recovery. One warning the doctor had given Gina was not to get pregnant, for at least five years. Pregnancy can activate hormones and precipitate a recurrence. Gina and Franklin had two children. Gina figured that was enough.

In 1997, Gina felt a large mass on the side of her stomach. She had Franklin feel it, just to make sure she wasn't imagining it. He felt it too and she promptly called the doctor. Her doctor ordered an ultrasound, which confirmed two things. Gina had a large fibroid tumor in her uterus and she was pregnant. After delivering a healthy baby girl, Gina underwent a full hysterectomy.

"The pregnancy must have stirred up something. In 2000, I was demonstrating how to perform a breast exam to a group of women at the American Cancer Society. I felt a small lump under my arm where I'd had the mastectomy. I thought it was probably nothing, but I called the doctor. He thought it was probably nothing, but told me to come in so he could be sure.

"We were both wrong. The results of the needle biopsy came back malignant. After ten years they don't call it a recurrence. They call it a new cancer. I don't know about that. It was in a little bit of breast tissue left after the mastectomy, and the cancer had spread to my lymph nodes.

"I called Franklin at work to tell him. He got really mad at me for not telling him right away, even though I thought it was nothing. I know he wasn't really mad. He was scared. His sister had died of breast cancer two years before. Now, he equated breast cancer with death.

"This time I had a lumpectomy, followed by chemotherapy. Before chemo I had my hair cut really short so I wouldn't freak out when it fell out. My mom and my older daughter, Pauline, came with me. They both had their hair cut really short in solidarity. It was really sweet.

"Six months of chemo were really horrible. But Franklin and the kids helped out a lot. My boss was great. He said, 'Come in when you can, leave if you feel bad.' I made it through."

As soon as she was able, Gina went back to volunteering at Reach Out to Recovery. "We were having a testimonial dinner at the Cancer Society. This woman, who I didn't recognize, was talking about how hard it had been for her getting breast cancer. Then she said one day an angel came to visit, listened to her story and answered her questions. After that she said she felt like she had the courage to go on. She pointed to me and said I was that angel.

"I was really touched, and embarrassed, because I didn't remember her. I see so many women. Just knowing I'd helped someone get through meant a lot to me. "I wish I could say that I felt like I was done with cancer. I'm expecting a third round. Things come in threes, you know. Franklin forbids me to talk like this. So, in front of him I don't.

"Having cancer has changed me. I speak up for myself. I haven't always been this outspoken," she winks slyly. "And I try to live my life to the fullest. I try new things. Last year I learned to ski and I love it.

"For the one-year anniversary of finishing treatment, Franklin and I celebrated by going on a Caribbean cruise. It was perfect. The days were sunny and the nights were warm. There I was dancing under the stars with my husband, wearing my strapless, emerald-green dress. Sometimes dreams do come true."

III

CANCER MADE ME GROW UP

NICOLE

AN EXPATRIATE AMERICAN COMES HOME

"I was 37 and living in Paris at the time. I reached up to get something down from a shelf and my arm brushed across my right breast. I thought I felt something unusual, so I examined my breast with my hand and found a good-sized lump.

"Part of me knew that I should go to see a doctor, but medicine in France is very different. Doctors are looked up to as gods and patients have no say in their treatment. Besides, I don't really believe in allopathic medicine. I decided to treat it through holistic medicine and work with alternative healers."

Nicole is a beautiful, biracial woman with milk-chocolate skin, oceanic blue eyes and a thick mane of brown curls. An artist by avocation and a romantic by disposition, she appears dreamy, almost ethereal.

She came to Paris drawn by the lore of the bohemian artists of the Left Bank in the early twentieth century. She attended college at the Sorbonne and stayed on after graduation, studying painting and working as an artist's model. She was living with her sculptor boyfriend, in the Marais district.

"I spent a year going to various alternative practitioners, acupuncturists, herbalists, homeopaths and even faith healers. The lump continued to grow. After a year, Jean Luc, my boyfriend, had had it. He insisted that I go to a doctor.

"I realized that I couldn't control this. I had to give up trying. When I finally did, it was really awful. The woman doctor who saw me was really mean. She hurt me performing the needle biopsy. When the results came back she told me that I had cancer and that it was my fault."

Nicole had an aggressive, 4 cm tumor with lymph node involvement. When she told Jean Luc, he immediately called his uncle, who was a doctor in Paris. His uncle said that if it were his girlfriend he'd send her back to the States, where medicine is a lot better.

Nicole called her parents in Los Angeles. Her father had a friend who was a doctor at the Mayo Clinic in Arizona. They made arrangements with the hospital and wired her the money for a plane ticket. Within a week, Nicole was on a plane to Arizona.

"The whole thing was surreal. The doctors examined me and told me that I'd have to have three months of chemotherapy before they could remove the tumor and for three months after. After the first chemo treatment all I did was sleep for two days, having one bizarre dream after another. Strange as it sounds, I felt like I'd been sent on this mysterious, perilous journey that was somehow necessary to move my life along to the next stage."

Nicole endured a horrible, three-month regime of chemotherapy, but was rewarded for her suffering. The tumor had shrunken by more than half and her lymph nodes were cancer-free.

After a month-long stay of execution, to have a lumpectomy and recover from the surgery, it was time to begin chemo again, followed by six weeks of radiation.

"I chose to go back to France for the second round of chemo. As miserable as the system was — waiting four or five hours for treatment, having them repeatedly lose my files, wondering if I'd be getting someone else's chemo treatment — it was free because of socialized medicine. I didn't have medical insurance. My parents paid for all the treatment at the Mayo Clinic. Having them pay any more just didn't seem fair.

"Two months after finishing radiation I was feeling pretty normal again. I wanted to do something symbolic of my cancer experience. I chose to make a pilgrimage. I hiked the Camino de Santiago to the

Cathedral de Santiago in Spain.

"This is a traditional pilgrimage, frequently associated with paying penance. It didn't feel that way to me. I know it sounds ridiculous, but I was consciously trying to duplicate the chemo experience. After each chemo session, no matter how terrible, no matter how much I didn't want to go back and do it again, the following week I was back there. I wanted to do something where I'd make a choice day after day to continue to do something until I'd reached my goal. For most of my life I'd quit doing things when the going got rough or I got bored.

"I hiked 400 kilometers, over 200 miles. There were days when I felt strong. There were other days where I felt so bad that I thought I just couldn't go on. But I did. I hiked at least 10 miles a day. When I reached the church I had one of the most profound experiences of my life, and I'm not even Catholic. I wept and wept, and thanked God for sparing my life in spite of me.

"It was at that point when I knew what I had to do next, and it was paying penance. I had to go home to the United States. I'd been living in Paris like this self-styled, bohemian fairy princess in Never Neverland. I romanticized the poverty until it got too tough, then I'd wire home and my parents would send bailout money. I needed to come home, pay my dues and begin my life as an adult.

"I had lived in France for so long, all of my adult life. Other than being fluent in the language, I felt like a foreigner in the country where I was born. I had to relearn the basics like using the phone and taking the bus.

"Instead of going back to Los Angeles, I moved to San Francisco. I rented an in-law studio apartment and took an entry-level, low-paying, social service job.

"My parents are both lawyers. As a child of privilege I went to private schools, college abroad. I never knew how the other half lived. Living in poverty in Paris was just playacting.

"Now I work with intravenous drug-users with HIV. My father is an educated, professional black man. Many of my clients are black men, too, but they haven't been so lucky in their lives. I can't say that I truly understand them. But because of the suffering that I went through with cancer, I have empathy and compassion for their suffering. When they tell me their stories, I really listen. Enduring suffering and being willing to fight back and reclaim your life earns anyone the right to be heard, in my book anyway.

"I'm going to start graduate school in the fall. I've been accepted into a master of social welfare program. When I finish the program I want to become a licensed clinical social worker. I'd like to work in a hospital setting with women in treatment for breast cancer and other reproductive cancers.

"I feel very grateful and I want to give something back. It took having breast cancer to get here. But, I've finally grown up and become an adult."

LORNAH

I'M NOT AS NICE, BUT I'M KINDER

Lornah was bubbling. Finally, at 45, she had met the right guy. He was charming, witty, very caring, and he was French. She was smitten. He popped the question. Without hesitation, she said yes.

There was a wrinkle. He was a single father of a 12-year-old daughter. Relocating to the States was out of the question. She would have to be willing to move to France. Lornah had never been to France, or had never wanted to go for that matter. She didn't speak the language. But, Lornah was a "good girl." She'd been raised to put the desires of others first. She never thought twice about her own needs when she agreed to move to France.

They would be moving a week after the wedding. Rather than chance dealing with a new medical system soon after moving, she scheduled all of her routine medical and dental exams before leaving.

She had a mammogram two weeks before the wedding. Soon after, she received a call from the doctor. He'd seen an irregularity on the film. He assured her that it was probably nothing. If she wasn't leaving he'd order another mammogram in six months. Since this wasn't possible, he asked Lornah to come in for a biopsy after the wedding, again emphasizing that it was probably nothing.

Three days after her wedding, she had the biopsy. The doctor found a malignancy. The good news was that it was ductile carcinoma in situ (DCIS): non-invasive, no nodal involvement. The bad news:

the tumor was large, 4 cm. The doctor recommended a mastectomy.

"I just couldn't do that to my husband, Henri," Lornah recalls. "There had to be another way."

She endured three surgeries in two months. It took two surgeries to get clear margins. The second surgery amounted to a partial mastectomy. The third surgery reduced her other D-cup breast to match.

Two weeks later, not having visibly recovered from her ordeal, she was on a plane heading for France, to start a new life with a new husband and a new family.

"It was awful," Lornah remembers. "I couldn't speak for myself, so my immune system spoke for me. It was as if I'd gone off to live in the most unsanitary place in the third world, without inoculations. I caught everything: colds, flu, freak infections.

"I was in a new country, where I didn't know anyone, didn't speak the language. The medical system is very different than it is here, very patronizing. They don't include the patient in the decision-making process, which for me, as a nurse, was infuriating.

"Henri's family was no help. They avoided me as much as possible. It was as if my recurring freak illness was somehow proof that I still had cancer. I think they were afraid if they got too close they might catch it.

"Henri, on the other hand, was wonderful. He took care of me, tried to keep my spirits up. One of my maladies was a middle-ear infection. I threw up so much I just carried a bowl around with me. He painted a picture of a clown on the bottom of the bowl. He kept me laughing through it all."

After about six months, Lornah's health stabilized and the doctors decided that she was ready to start radiation.

"What a reward. I had been so isolated, just me, Henri and his daughter Sophie. When I started radiation I met another woman who'd had breast cancer. I realized how alone I'd felt with the disease. I remember just hugging her and crying.

"Radiation was horrible. The skin over my breast burned and peeled after every treatment, like some hideous sunburn. My skin was so raw I couldn't tolerate wearing a bra. But I still had to go back the next day and have it done to me again. I assumed that this is what every woman goes through and that my six-month health ordeal had turned me into a wimp.

"After the last treatment, the doctor told me that I had had the worst reaction she'd ever seen. She didn't tell me before, because she figured I'd quit. I wouldn't have. She robbed me of the opportunity to feel brave, instead of feeling like a wimp."

When Lornah regained her health, she started exploring her new home and meeting people. She enrolled in a language school and started learning French. Finally she was ready to start her new life. Unfortunately, a nasty twist had been waiting just out of view.

She knew that Henri had had a history of depression when she married him. She had never evidenced it in their too-brief courtship and was more than willing to relegate it to the past. She figured that love conquers all. It didn't. The strain of Lornah's illness had proved too much for him. As soon as she recovered, he fell apart and had to be hospitalized.

"After he got out of the hospital he was on a lot of medication: too much medication, the wrong medication, I didn't know. I just knew that it didn't work. He was suicidal. We had a plate-glass door on our shower. He'd talk about throwing himself through it or hanging himself on the equipment where he worked at the technical college.

"I felt like I couldn't even afford to go to sleep. I had to watch him all of the time. I couldn't leave him at home if I had to go to the store. But, I couldn't take him into the store. He might be overwhelmed and have a panic attack. So, I'd leave him in the car, run into the store, run back out and take him home."

Eventually, he stabilized enough that Lornah could go out and leave him at home. He was even able to go back to work. The structure seemed to help him. But things were still far from right.

About that time, he went into a new phase. "He stopped talking to me," Lornah recalls. "I'd ask him a question and he wouldn't respond. We'd go weeks like that. I couldn't have anyone over, because it might overstimulate him and bring on a panic attack. So it was just Sophie and I, walking around on eggshells. Occasionally Henri would flip out, then he'd go back to being mute. We'd been married for three years and I thought, 'I can't go on like this or I'll be suicidal.'"

Lornah's "way out" came soon after. She got a call from a health organization she'd worked for stateside. They'd received a six-month grant for a new project and they wanted her to work on it. She gratefully accepted.

Henri's brother and sister-in-law could come and stay with Henri and Sophie, so she didn't have to worry about them. She called her friend Jill, in California, who was thrilled to have Lornah coming back home. Jill's neighbor had a guest cottage that she was willing to rent to Lornah for a nominal amount. It began to look like things were falling into place nicely.

The night before her departure, Lornah was so excited she couldn't sleep. The next morning she went over her list of instructions with her sister-in-law, kissed Henri and Sophie goodbye, and called a cab to take her to De Gaulle Airport.

"After the plane took off I felt this enormous sense of relief, as if a huge weight had been lifted. I felt that I'd earned this time away. I'd go back home for six months, recharge my batteries, and come back better than ever, able to handle the situation. I felt so good I treated myself to a glass of wine."

Hours later the plane landed at San Francisco International Airport. Jill was waiting to meet her. She saw Jill and ran to hug her. Jill barely recognized her. She hadn't seen Lornah since the wedding. She knew all about France, and expected it to show, but not this much.

"It was a little unnerving," Jill recalls. "At first I didn't even recognize Lornah. She was so thin and pale. She's always seemed so fit and healthy. But it was more than that. It was like her body was still here, coming home, but her soul had been sucked out of her.

"I was back for about three weeks," Lornah remembers. "I woke up one morning and was shocked to realize that I felt normal. I hadn't realized it, but I'd been unhappy and depressed for so long I'd forgotten what normal felt like. It was at that moment that it finally hit me. I had to leave my marriage and come back home.

"Before cancer, I would have said Henri and Sophie need me too much. I can wait to be happy, someday. After cancer, I've learned that someday may never come. I have a responsibility to Henri and Sophie. But more importantly, I have a responsibility to myself and my own happiness."

After the grant ended, Lornah went back to France. She told Henri that she planned to move back to the States. He pleaded with her, promised to go to therapy, take his medicine, anything to keep her. He tried for awhile, but ultimately sunk back into his helpless, hopeless state again.

"Leaving Henri was the easy part. Leaving Sophie was tough. I really love her. I love being a mom, and I'm good at it. If I'd known, I would have had my own children in my 30s. But now I had Sophie and she needed me. Her birth mother was manic-depressive and abusive. Between her mother and her father, Sophie had never had much of a chance.

"I had promised to help her get into a college preparatory high school, and I planned to keep my promise. She loves animals and wants to be a veterinarian. She's a bright kid. With a little help I think she can make it.

"I stayed for another year and a half. Sophie got into the high school. I taught Henri how to cook, clean and handle finances. I realized that my having done everything hadn't helped him learn to help himself. I accepted my responsibility and when I finally left I had no guilt. It was my turn, finally.

"The first year without me was rough for them. But they made it, and they're both a lot more independent and self-confident for it. I go back to France once a year and Sophie comes here to spend the summer with me. She is truly the gift of my marriage. I never really had a husband, but I now have a daughter, and always will.

"Cancer changed me a lot. I'm not as nice as I used to be, but I'm kinder. I used to be a pushover, always trying to please other people, at my expense. Now I stand up for myself and some people don't like it. I've lost a few friends. My mother still hasn't forgiven me for leaving Henri. Others say they like me better and have a lot more respect for me. More important, I've come to respect myself.

"Cancer has made me better at my job. I'm a public health nurse. I visit people in their homes. It's not like taking care of someone for a few days in a hospital. I develop long-term relationships with my patients. I ask them how they feel about their illness, how it affects their families. I'm not afraid to tell them that I had cancer. People seem to find enormous relief in finally being able to talk about what's going on.

"I can say, maybe for the first time in my life, that I'm happy, really happy. I used to think that happiness was something you had to earn: do enough good deeds, earn enough 'good girl green stamps,' and I'd be worthy of happiness. Or, I thought it was something you seek, marry the right man and he'd make me happy. I know now that it's not a place to try to get to, but a place to realize that I already am. Buddhists say, 'Happiness isn't having what you want, but wanting what you have.' I do."

IV

NO MORE FUN HOUSE MIRRORS

TRUDIE

I'M NOT MY MOTHER

"My life was just getting back to normal. I'd been on and off, mostly on disability for ten years for chronic fatigue and environmental illnesses. My marriage had fallen apart. I'd gone through bankruptcy. Finally it was behind me and I was back at work.

"Environmental illness makes a social pariah of you. I was allergic to everything: car exhaust, cigarette smoke, paint fumes, pesticides. Going anywhere was like walking through a minefield, never knowing when one would explode. Eventually I just stopped going out altogether.

"The way people treat you is just awful. I was called a hypochondriac, told that I should see a psychiatrist. I gave up on mainstream medicine and only went to see alternative practitioners. At least they really believed that I was sick.

"Anyway, it was the dawning of the new millennium and thankfully all that health stuff was behind me. Or so I thought."

Trudie had gone for her annual OB-GYN exam. The doctor felt a lump on the left breast. She ordered a mammogram and referred Trudie to a surgeon.

"The mammogram came back clear. The surgeon could feel the lump, but told me that it was probably a cyst, nothing to worry about. I was 55 at the time and postmenopausal. How could I have a cyst? I was on hormone replacement. I convinced myself that that must be causing it. I was ready to believe anything that would tell me that I wasn't sick again."

The following year, Trudie's gynecologist felt the same lump. This time it felt bigger. She sent Trudie back to the surgeon, who ordered a mammogram and an ultrasound. Both came back clear.

"This time I wasn't going for this cyst business. I planned to get a second opinion and get to the bottom of it."

Trudie's plans were swiftly derailed. She'd been hobbling around on an arthritic knee for several years. Her orthopedist told her that she needed knee replacement surgery now, before things got any worse.

With trepidation, Trudie consented to surgery. Then things got worse. After surgery, while still in the hospital, Trudie contracted a staph infection and her already compromised immune system went berserk.

She spent six months in the hospital. She couldn't stomach the food and her weight dropped to a scrawny 90 pounds. Her skin hung like an empty sack from her frame. She became addicted to morphine, detoxed, and went through withdrawals. The doctors walked a tightrope to give her enough pain medicine to take the edge off the constant, excruciating pain, and not re-addict her.

After recovering from the knee ordeal, Trudie went back to the surgeon to check on the lump. Now even the surgeon thought that it was bigger. She ordered another mammogram and ultrasound. This time, both showed an irregularity. A needle biopsy proved the irregularity to be malignant.

"It turns out that I had lobular breast cancer, which accounts for only 5% to 15% of all cases of breast cancer, depending on who you ask. It can't be detected on either a mammogram or an ultrasound until it's pretty far gone. I was beside myself knowing that I'd been walking around with cancer all that time. I just kept thinking about my mother.

"My mother was diagnosed with breast cancer when she was 55, just like me. It didn't kill her. I think she'd been better off if it had. Her life just started to deteriorate afterwards. She'd always been a loud, boisterous person. After cancer, she just withdrew and withered. She was seriously depressed. She wouldn't eat and lost a lot of weight.

I guess she had osteoporosis because she started shrinking. She looked like a shriveled-up old witch. Between 55 and 65, she had three heart attacks. The last one killed her. I was terrified that I'd been cursed to repeat her fate."

Trudie had a lumpectomy. The doctor removed a large, 3.5 cm tumor. Then, she waited, breathless, for two weeks for her results. The doctor delivered the good news and the bad news. There was no lymph node involvement. But they didn't get clear margins. Another surgery would be necessary.

"One of the best things that I did after I was diagnosed was to join a breast cancer support group. They kept me going through the tough times: the waiting and not knowing, the bad news. When the surgeon told me that she didn't get all of the cancer, I'd had it with her. What I needed from my group were referrals to other surgeons.

"Group members provided me with a few names. My friend Geri gave me the name of her surgeon, who was quite esteemed in the cancer community. She also offered to go with me on my first visit. I agreed and made an appointment.

"The doctor seemed okay at first. She examined me and ordered an MRI to get a better look at the tumor, or what was left of it. But then she started interrogating me. Was I Jewish? I said yes. Was I Ashkenazi? I said yes. Then she told me I was very high risk and should seriously consider having a bilateral mastectomy.

"I left in shock. I'm glad that Geri came with me. But one thing that I knew for sure was that I didn't want to see the doctor again. I decided to try another group member's referral.

"Surgeon number three was a kindly, gentle man. He said that he would order a copy of my MRI for himself. He didn't want to be hasty in making a recommendation until he had all the facts. Leaving his office, I felt a lot better."

When the results of the MRI came back, Trudie went back to see the third surgeon. "He told me that based on the MRI, my tumor, or at least what was left of it, was so large that he would recommend my having chemotherapy before surgery to shrink the tumor. As someone with a history of environmental illness, chemotherapy terrified me. I was having no part of this.

"I left his office shell-shocked. Thinking that I could trust him, I'd come to the appointment alone. Now I felt like my brain was in quicksand. I felt unsafe driving home."

As Trudie slowly headed home, her cell phone rang. It was the second surgeon, who had also received the results of the MRI. She said that the results looked good. All that would be needed was another lumpectomy.

"It never occurred to me to question how two esteemed surgeons could come up with such divergent takes on the same test results. All I knew was that one recommended chemotherapy, while the other said that all I needed was a lumpectomy. I scheduled the surgery."

The second surgery still failed to produce clear margins and Trudie underwent a mastectomy.

"After the mastectomy I sort of flipped out," she recalls. "I just wasn't healing. I was exhausted all of the time. I had shortness of breath and heart palpitations. I went to the emergency room twice with chest pains.

"One night I was lying in bed and I couldn't sleep. This feeling of impending doom rushed over me. Then the left side of my chest started to ache, not the skin, but deep in my chest. I was sweating and breathing rapidly. I called 911.

"The ER doctor said that I wasn't having a heart attack. The pain was probably just nerves that had been cut in surgery regenerating. The sweating and rapid breathing sounded more like a panic attack. He gave me a prescription for Valium and told me that I should see a psychiatrist."

When Trudie recounted the story, group members could empathize and support her. The leader, Vickie, broached the subject of Trudie's need for therapy more tactfully.

She told Trudie that the stress of cancer frequently causes old issues to surface and become problematic. Many survivors find individual therapy helpful at this time. Several group members agreed, saying that they were in therapy now themselves and found it invaluable. After the group ended, Trudie asked Vickie for a referral.

"Vickie referred me to Sara, a breast cancer survivor herself, who specializes in working with survivors. I liked Sara immediately, and wished it hadn't taken me so long to find her.

"Sara suggested that I was over-identifying with my mother and expected her fate to be my fate. She wondered why. I remembered when my mother had breast cancer I wasn't very sympathetic. I was in my 30s, and on my own. Besides, my relationship with my mother had always been a difficult one. She cursed me for my lack of compassion and said that when I got breast cancer I would understand and be sorry.

"Sara seemed appalled and asked if I remembered anything like that from my childhood. At first I said no. But, then I remembered that when I was about 10, my mother was in bed with a migraine. I guess I wasn't saying or doing the right thing because she told me that she hoped I'd get migraines someday so I'd understand how she felt. My mother was the worst kind of Jewish mother, a real guilt provoker. Sure enough, by my 20s I was getting migraines on a regular basis.

"Sara said that it looked like I had accepted my mother's ill health as my legacy. I didn't have to accept that. I had a choice. I wasn't my mother.

"At first I thought that was the most ridiculous thing I'd ever heard. It was like Sara was saying that my mother had put a curse on me and I'd accepted it. But gradually I started to realize that there was a grain of truth in it. I'd had a lot of illness in my life and that was real. But I'd identified myself with illness and let it limit my life. I decided that I'd had enough of that. Maybe there's heart disease or who knows what down the line for me, but it's not here now. Why borrow trouble?

"After that I slowly started feeling better. I never had another heart attack scare or panic attack," she laughs. "It took breast cancer to teach me that I'm not a sick person after all."

CELESTE

I THOUGHT I WAS THE POSTER CHILD FOR BREAST CANCER IN RECOVERY

"I had my first bout with breast cancer in 1990, when I was only 46. I had ductile carcinoma in situ (DCIS). It was being hotly debated at the time whether DCIS was cancer or just a precancerous condition.

"Anyway, I had a lumpectomy and radiation. They gave me thirty-five radiation treatments that were much stronger than they feel are safe to give today. I didn't know that at the time. I only knew that they made me feel sick, tired and fluish all the time."

Celeste barely had enough time to have cancer. Divorced a year earlier, she had to support herself for the first time in her life. She was working in sales, taking real estate classes at night.

"I spent my recovery time studying for the real estate licensing exam, which I passed shortly after radiation was done."

It was the early nineties and the real estate boom was just getting started. A self-acknowledged overachiever, Celeste found herself working ten- to twelve-hour days, six to seven days a week. Caught up in the whirlwind of her new career, she left the experience of cancer behind her.

"I met a woman who had breast cancer and was having a hard time. It never occurred to me to tell her that I was a breast cancer survivor. Was I in denial or what?" Celeste had remarried and was successful in her career. Her life appeared to be humming along nicely.

Then in 2000 she noticed, or thought she noticed, changes in her right breast.

"I kept checking my breast. I thought it looked different, but I wasn't sure. I had a scar from the surgery and skin changes from the radiation, so it looked different from the other one anyway. I even asked my husband, Sid, if he thought it looked different. Since neither of us were sure, I decided to wait and see.

"Then one morning when I checked my breast, my nipple was white. Then I was scared. I made an appointment with my surgeon. He extracted some fluid and sent it to the lab. The results came back positive. I had breast cancer, again.

"I was in shock. Sure, I kept checking and I went to the doctor when the nipple changed. But I expected it to be nothing. It wasn't nothing. It was cancer."

It turned out to be lobular breast cancer, a rare form of breast cancer that accounts for only about 15% of all cases and tends to be detected later in the disease's progression. It had spread throughout Celeste's breast. A lumpectomy wouldn't be an option this time. She needed to have a mastectomy.

"I was beside myself knowing that I'd have to have a mastectomy. It was two weeks before the surgery was scheduled and I kind of flipped out. I kept going to Home Depot, buying plants and planting them in the garden. I went on a cleaning binge, cleaning the house top to bottom. When I was done I'd start over again. I got obsessed with all the fibers in the carpet going the same way, so I kept vacuuming over and over. I painted the kitchen and the bathroom." Her husband and friends just watched in amazement. But, nobody dared say anything.

Celeste had her surgery and waited for the results. "The worst part of breast cancer isn't the surgery or radiation or even chemotherapy. It's waiting for the results. It's like getting suspended in midair. You can't touch down until you know what's next.

"The nurse called me and made an appointment to see the doctor for my results. It wasn't good news. The doctor got dirty margins, in other words, he didn't get all of the cancer. How could he do a mastectomy and not get all of the cancer?"

The cancer had spread from Celeste's breast to her pectoralis muscle. The treatment of choice was either surgery or radiation. The surgeon wanted to remove the muscle, fearing that more radiation could damage Celeste's heart or lungs. The radiologist wanted to do radiation, reasoning that surgery could leave her incapacitated. The surgeon won. Meanwhile, Celeste fell apart.

"I couldn't eat. I couldn't sleep. I'd just shake involuntarily. The doctor put me on antidepressants and wrote me a prescription for Valium. I took them occasionally to sleep but I hated the idea of being on drugs all the time to get through this.

"The women in my support group made me a poster with my picture in the middle and all their pictures in a circle around it. It read, 'We're all walking with you.' Between repeatedly looking at my poster, going to my support group and doing creative visualizations three times a day, I survived the month between the mastectomy and the removal of my pectoralis muscle."

Results of the second surgery brought more bad news. The cancer had spread to Celeste's chest wall. Now she would need chemotherapy, followed by more radiation.

"This time I completely lost it. I had to go to the lab to have my blood drawn. Fortunately, Sid was with me. I was shaking so hard that Sid had to hold me down while the technician drew my blood. This time my attitude about getting through was, 'Screw it, I'll take the drugs.'"

Celeste endured four excruciating rounds of chemotherapy. With the help of Sid and her support group, she made it through. Then she had to face radiation. "Radiation terrified me. I think that radiation caused the second cancer. How could I possibly believe that it could cure it?

"The kinder, gentler radiation turned out to be nothing in comparison with the stuff I'd had before. The best thing was that all the radiation put together didn't do my heart any damage. There was a little damage to my right lung, but it was minimal."

In her recovery, Celeste's overachieving instincts went into high gear. She switched to an organic, macrobiotic diet, started practicing yoga for an hour a day and meditation for another hour.

"Everything was going great. Yoga was bringing mobility back to my arm and shoulder that was far more than the doctor had ever expected. I'd lost 20 pounds through my ordeal. Now I was eating so well that I was healthier and looking better than I had in years. Most importantly, I was feeling this kind of inner peace.

"Then September 11 happened. I was glued to the TV watching the news. I kept seeing the Twin Towers crumble, over and over again. I started to go into stress mode, like all of it was happening to me. I couldn't eat. I couldn't sleep. I started catching whatever bug was going around."

Celeste called Linda, who'd been the leader of her support group. Linda listened to Celeste's plight and suggested that they work together in individual psychotherapy.

Initially, Linda intervened behaviorally. She asked Celeste not to watch the news or read pertinent sections of the newspaper for two weeks. Then she could gradually add them back in, but only within her tolerance limits. If the news upset her she needed to turn off the TV or put down the paper.

In therapy they explored the cause of Celeste's distress. Celeste kept equating the terrorist attacks with cancer. For her the attacks had become personal. Just when she felt safe from the cancer recurring, the terrorist attacks happened. She panicked. They made her feel out of control. She couldn't protect herself.

Although Celeste had seen her new, "super-healthy" lifestyle as making her a poster child for breast cancer in recovery, she had created an obsessively healthy lifestyle as a sort of talisman. She believed that if she could construct a healthy enough lifestyle she would be immune. Cancer could never invade her again. The terrorist attacks foiled her plan. Unconsciously, she had equated the terrorist attacks with cancer. Her hermetically sealed lifestyle had not made her impenetrable to attack. Without the illusion of her newly constructed defenses, she panicked.

"It took a long time. I guess I was pretty resistant at first. But slowly I started to realize there was really no way I could protect myself from a recurrence. It was great that I'd cleaned up my act and had a healthy lifestyle. But I got a little carried away."

Celeste was able to relax a little. Though she still tries to buy organic, she dropped the ultra-limiting macrobiotic plan in favor of a more varied plant-based diet. She even started allowing herself an occasional dessert or glass of wine.

"One really great thing came out of my obsessive phase," she laughs. "Yoga. It's given me more mobility than I ever would have dreamed. I'm studying to become a yoga teacher and work with breast cancer survivors.

"But I didn't want to wait to give something back. I've become a peer counselor at the breast health center. I meet newly diagnosed women, and listen to their stories. I hear their fears, their anger, and their denial. I know it all. I've been there.

"I'll be 60 next month. Sid is taking me to Paris to celebrate. It's the one place I've always wanted to go. With all that rich food and wine, to say nothing of secondhand smoke, I could never have handled being there in my macrobiotic phase," she laughs.

"I still plan to avoid secondhand smoke as much as possible. But I plan to enjoy the food and wine. I've had to accept that I can't prevent a recurrence. But I can try to enjoy my life and live it to the fullest now, and let the future happen as it happens."

V

THE WOUNDED HEALERS

RUTH

AIN'T NO MOUNTAIN HIGH ENOUGH

"I was in shock. I tried to go on with my life as usual. I went to my psychotherapy office on Tuesday, planning to see my clients. I made it through two sessions and realized that I couldn't do it. I cancelled the rest of the sessions for the week.

"My husband, Lou, took me out to lunch at a place near my office. We were sitting on the patio, watching people go by: moms pushing their babies in strollers, kids on skateboards, UPS drivers double-parking their brown trucks to make a delivery. Their lives were going on as usual. But ours couldn't. It was as if we were separate, encapsulated by cancer."

Just the day before, Ruth had gone to her OB-GYN for her yearly checkup. The doctor found a small lump in her right breast, though her recent mammogram had been clear.

"I wasn't worried. There was no breast cancer in my family. I was 47, which I somehow rationalized was too young to have cancer."

Her doctor wasn't much more concerned than Ruth, but elected to perform a needle biopsy, just to be sure. The results came back malignant.

The doctor referred her to a surgeon in the building. Fortunately, the surgeon had a cancellation, and could see Ruth that afternoon.

"My oldest daughter was picking me up after my appointment. She said that she knew from the moment she saw me walking towards the car that something was wrong, very wrong.

"I got into the car and told her that I had cancer. We held each other, and we both cried. She cancelled her appointments for the afternoon and went to the surgeon's office with me."

The surgery was scheduled for that Friday. Ruth tried to go on with business as usual, and learned quickly that that wasn't going to work. Instead she spent hours in the breast center's library, immersing herself in as much breast cancer literature as she could tolerate.

"I don't know if it helped. One minute I'd find something that scared the hell out of me, the next I'd find something reassuring. I think the real point was having something to occupy my mind, to keep me from going nuts worrying."

The day of the surgery, Lou and both daughters accompanied her to the hospital. She was having a lumpectomy, surgery done on an outpatient basis. Ruth's family would be taking her back home later that day. They set up a task schedule, to take care of her and keep the house running over the weekend.

By Monday, everyone had gone back to work. Ruth waited at home, alone, for the doctor to call with the results.

"I was really nervous," Ruth recalled. "I knew, whatever the outcome was, that I could handle it. It was the not knowing that was killing me. I took a pain pill, then had a glass of wine, something I would normally never do."

The surgeon called around 4:00 with the good news. She'd removed a 5 cm tumor, with clean margins. There was no lymph node involvement. Six weeks of radiation was all that would be required.

Ruth wept with relief. Then she called her husband and daughters with the good news.

"I was very fortunate to have gotten off so easily, and I'm grateful. I knew, even so, that I didn't want to drift back into business as usual, and forget that cancer ever happened. I wanted to do something. I just didn't know what."

Ruth found that in her psychotherapy practice, both new and long-term clients seemed to be dealing with life-threatening illness in themselves or those close to them. Her own experience helped her to be more empathetic and helpful to her clients. But it wasn't enough.

Ruth went to a breast cancer fundraiser. There, she met some women from the Breast Cancer Fund, a group that organizes hikes and peak climbs to raise money to fund investigations into the role that environmental factors play in the development of breast cancer.

Ruth signed up for an upcoming seven-mile hike with trepidation. "I wanted to help and I wanted to participate. I walk and do yoga, but I'd never been athletic. Secretly, I think that I was afraid that I couldn't do it."

Ruth raised $500. "The day of the hike, I was almost as nervous as I was the day of my surgery. The hike was tough and I was definitely one of the 'slow ones,' but I made it." She was thrilled, and immediately signed up for another hike.

The Breast Cancer Fund was planning a peak climb in six months. They'd be climbing Mount Shasta. The 14,162-foot climb would take three days. The Fund would provide training and equipment. The climber would be required to raise $10,000.

Her friends from the Fund encouraged Ruth to sign up. "The thought of it initially scared me to death. But I've always had this alter ego I've never told anyone about. She's this athletic woman who backpacks. I'd completed a few hikes by then and was in the best shape I'd ever been in my life. More importantly, I'd survived breast cancer. I figured that I owed it to myself to give this a try."

The training hikes were grueling. On several occasions, Ruth had been tempted to give up.

On one long hike, Ruth and two other slow hikers had fallen behind and were in jeopardy of losing the group. Pam, one of the strongest hikers in the group, got worried. She dropped back and found the stragglers. She hiked along with them, encouraging them as they went, until they all finished, well after dark.

Pam remembers, "It was our second training hike and far too difficult for us at that point. Most of us were marathon runners and triathletes. We bitched like crazy. Ruth was the least fit of all of us, and she never complained. I thought that she must have gone through so much, having cancer, that this hardship was nothing in comparison. From that day on, Ruth was my hero."

On another hike, Ruth remembers being the only one left at the back of the pack. "I was climbing up this steep cliff and I kept beating myself up, telling myself that I was an idiot to have ever gotten into this — that I should just give up now and not be a burden to the group.

"Then I heard a voice that managed to out-scream my inner critic. She said, 'Look how far you've come. You've done things you'd never believed you could have. Why can't you make it to the summit of Mount Shasta?' From then on, slow or not, I knew I'd make it."

As the day of the climb neared, Ruth, with the well wishes of her family and friends, packed her bags and drove her Honda to Mount Shasta.

She spent the night before the climb at a motel where several other climbers were staying. They met in one of the women's rooms. "We were all so excited, like teenage girls at a slumber party: talking, laughing, getting way too little sleep."

The next day, the group climbed to their base camp at 7,880 feet. Here, they learned how to use the crampons and ice axes they would need to ascend the frozen slopes to the summit before dawn the next day.

Ruth was awakened the next morning at 1:00. With her headlamp turned on and her ice axe and trekking poles, she started on the long trudge to the summit.

Of the 48 climbers who began that day, only 14 would reach the summit. Ruth was not one of them. At 10,000 feet, she experienced the headache and lightheaded giddiness symptomatic to altitude sickness.

"I don't mind not summating. When I reached Helen Lake, I was very giddy and disoriented. The leader felt that it would have been dangerous for me to go on, even if I took altitude-sickness medicine.

"But I reached my own summit, accomplishing something I would never have dreamed of attempting before. I felt no disappointment or regret."

Since her peak climb, Ruth and Lou have gone on several backpacking trips which they've thoroughly enjoyed.

"This summer I tried rock climbing, and loved it. I've been running and cycling, too. I think I'd like to try a triathlon. I can hardly believe it, but I've become the woman of my dreams. Without breast cancer, I would never have had the guts to try."

KATE

DEFYING THE LEGACY

Kate stumbled through the front door, arms weighed down with shopping bags. She had a bottle of Dom Perignon, a tin of beluga caviar, a hunk of French Brie, a baguette and a large bouquet of flowers. Heaving a sigh of relief, she laid her bounty to rest on the kitchen counter. She picked up the phone and called Paul, her husband of almost thirty years, at his law office. "Be home early, we're having a celebration," was the cryptic message she left on his voice mail.

As she put the bottle of champagne in the refrigerator and found a vase for the flowers, she thought, "A celebration indeed." Today she was 51 years, 5 months and 1 day old. And she had outlived her mother.

Kate's mother had lost her six-year battle with breast cancer when she was 51 years, 5 months, to the day. Kate's sister, Jane, had died of the disease at 47. Her maternal grandmother had also died of it.

For as long as she could remember, Kate had oscillated between two diametrically opposed mind states: the grim acceptance that she, too, would get breast cancer and inevitably die of it by middle age; and a "the hell I will, I've still got a lot more living to do" attitude. But for today, the celebration of life was the order of the day.

Kate is a petite dynamo of a woman, with a silky, chestnut pageboy and luminous blue eyes. With Ralph Lauren Country style, the complete absence of pretension and a gentle but firm directness, she projects a Betty Ford kind of energy. But, like other women of her generation, Kate was raised to look after the needs of others and not burden them with her problems. The time built up anticipating her twice-yearly clinical breast exams and yearly mammogram were her own private hell.

Without her saying anything, though, Paul somehow knew. She and Paul had a ritual. After her exam she would immediately call him at the office. He would ask, "How did it go?" She would answer with a reassuring, "Just fine." She'd hear a sigh of relief. Then they'd both laugh.

Everything changed the year she turned 59. She'd had a clean mammogram a few months earlier, but in her clinical breast exam the doctor felt something. Kate said, "My heart sank into my toes, because I knew it was cancer." The doctor put Kate's hand on the lump and asked if she could feel it. She couldn't.

She was sent down the hall for another mammogram. Again, the results were negative. "Still," said the doctor, "I won't be able to sleep tonight if I don't get a sonogram." Again, Kate was sent down the hall. This time she was given an appointment for four days later.

She made the ritual call to Paul. "How did it go?" he asked. She hesitated for a moment. "Just fine." He heard it in her voice. "Something's wrong. I'm coming right home."

"Don't they realize what it does to someone, making them wait for four days, not knowing?" she asked. In four days, Kate's mind raced ahead four years. The tumor was, of course, malignant, and aggressive at that. It would metastasize to the lungs. First, there would be shortness of breath on stairs and hills, then just walking would be laborious, and finally, oxygen would be required to make breathing possible at all. Then there would be the brain metastasis: first, the occasional searing headache; then vertigo and blurred vision; finally, the loss of sight altogether.

Needless to say, four days later Kate was a wreck. Paul had to accompany her to the sonogram. The sonogram showed a mass. She was sent for a needle biopsy. The biopsy came back malignant.

As Kate went from room to room, test to test, doctor to doctor, she was grateful to have Paul along taking notes. She felt so shell-shocked, she'd walk out of each room remembering nothing that had been said. She and Paul met with her surgeon to discuss treatment options. She would have a lumpectomy with radiation or a mastectomy. The surgeon gave them a few days to think about it, discuss it and make their decision.

Since they live within walking distance of the medical center, Kate declined Paul's offer of a ride home, feeling the walk would help to clear her head. Sending Paul back to his office, Kate started home. "I remember walking through my own neighborhood like I was sleep-walking through a dream. At one point, I felt so overwhelmed I just sat down on someone's stairs and started to cry. This cat, who appeared to belong to the owner of the house, came towards me. She let me stroke her and cuddle her. I just sat there crying, cuddling the cat, talking to the cat. Finally, I pulled myself together and walked home. I still see that cat in the neighborhood. I'm still grateful to her."

Kate, Paul and their children discussed the treatment options. Kate decided on a mastectomy. "I'm not going to be nursing any more babies. Why not just take the breast and be done with it? While they're at it, why not just take them both?

Kate quickly learned that requesting a bilateral mastectomy was easier said than done. Doctors kept asking her if she was sure. Had she really taken enough time to think about it? They even required her to meet with the psychiatrist to evaluate whether she was an appropriate candidate for bilateral mastectomy.

"I was sitting in the psychiatrist's office. She was asking me questions and making notes on her clipboard." Kate recalled, "She got a call on her cell phone. She said it was an emergency and would I excuse her for a few minutes? I said of course.

"After she left the room I looked at the clipboard. By the time I was 10, like everyone else, I had learned to read upside down. I figured out where this was going and how to answer. When the psychiatrist came back I answered all of her questions correctly. She said she thought that I was an excellent candidate for a bilateral mastectomy and would tell my surgeon."

The date for her surgery was set for three weeks later. This gave Kate's anxiety a running start. "I tried to act like a warrior preparing for battle: calm, rational," she remembered. "The warrior act with cancer is such a front. I was scared to death, but I couldn't bring myself to tell anyone.

"In the family we were all playacting too. Someone would say, 'Don't worry, everything will be fine,' and we'd all agree. We were all tiptoeing around the proverbial elephant in the living room. No one was willing to be the first to admit it."

In the meantime, Kate and Paul had to go back East for a family wedding. The whole flight, Kate kept herself turned towards the window, sobbing softly. "I kept thinking, 'I'm going to die. I wonder which one of these beautiful flight attendants my husband will end up marrying.'"

When Kate returned home, she told the story to her support group. The leader reassured her that as improbable a situation as it was, it was a common fantasy of married women in the early stages of breast cancer.

At this point, Kate wasn't even ready to open up to her support group (something she laughs at in retrospect). Fortunately, her closest friend of almost fifty years, Pat, had flown into town to be with her.

"We went out to lunch and each of us had a couple of glasses of wine, something I almost never do. It must have loosened both of us up, because I blurted out, 'I'm scared, really scared, more scared than I've ever been in my life.' Then I cried. She said that she was scared, and cried too. There we were, both of us crying right there in the restaurant. We must have been a sight."

Fortunately, Pat, a clinical psychologist, was able to put her professional hat on at just the right moment. She asked Kate what she was afraid of. Kate said, "Dying."

"That's not it," Pat said. "I've known you almost fifty years. You love life more than anyone I know. You're not afraid of dying. You're afraid that your love affair with life is going to be cut short, before you're ready."

They both cried, then laughed, then cried.

Before the surgery, Kate's son and daughter had both flown in and were staying with their parents. The day of the surgery, at 5:30 in the morning, the four of them walked down to the hospital together.

Kate went through pre-op and was lying on the gurney, ready to go into surgery. The old terror returned. She kept insisting, "I'm going to die, I'm going to die."

"You can't die," snapped her daughter, Claire. "You haven't taught me how to make crêpes suzette yet."

It was like having a slap of cold water in her face. Kate calmed right down and was fine after that.

Kate's surgery was deemed a success. She recovered fairly quickly. With the help of her family and her support group, she began to put her life back together.

"I've become a much more emotional person," she said. "Life is so fragile. I feel other people's pain so much more. And I don't sweat the small stuff. It doesn't bother me if I can't find a parking place, or what the weather's like. I'm more honest about my feelings, too. I don't deliberately hurt people's feelings. But I'm not afraid to call it as I see it."

One rough spot to be gotten over in her recovery was sex. Paul, a prostate cancer survivor, needed to use Viagra to perform. Kate worried that her breastless body would only make matters worse.

They decided to deal with the issue ceremoniously and travel to one of their favorite romantic spots in Mexico. Beforehand, Paul made an appointment for the two of them with a counselor at Good Vibrations, a women's sex novelty store. The tattooed, body-pierced, twentysomething counselor provided them with a "toy box" of marital aids and explained various uses. "We had a ball," Kate recalls. With his Viagra, her mastectomy swimsuit (complete with falsies) and their box of toys, they were off to Mexico.

"What we learned," Kate said, "is that sex isn't about body parts. It's about the intimate connection shared by two people. Cancer can't take that away."

Kate's recovery went well for two years, then disaster appeared to strike. Kate caught a cold she couldn't seem to shake. It worsened into some sort of respiratory infection that didn't respond to antibiotics. Since Kate was a breast cancer survivor, her doctor ordered a CAT scan, just to rule out a lung metastasis. What it showed was a spot on her lung.

Because it was only one spot, not several, the doctor opted for surgery instead of chemotherapy. "Whatever it is, I want it out," he told her.

Kate revisited her old terrors. "It's cancer and I'm going to die." The last two years hadn't been a rebirth only a stay of execution. Again, Kate found herself lying on a gurney, waiting to go into surgery. She remembers vividly, "I didn't know if there was a God. But, just in case, I prayed, 'Just get me through this mess and I promise to give something back, something important.'"

Kate came through surgery well, again. She was resting in her room, with her family around her. The surgeon brought the results up himself. A piece had been removed from her lung and it was benign. Kate, Paul and their children wept with relief and gratitude.

When Kate had sufficiently recovered, she kept her promise. She signed up with the breast cancer center as a volunteer peer counselor. She would meet with women soon after their diagnoses. She would help them sort through the voluminous information available so they could make informed decisions. She offered a hand to hold, a shoulder to cry on, and when needed, a "slap of cold water in the face."

Peer counseling alone wasn't enough for Kate. She looked for other ways to help. She remembered long hours spent in waiting rooms to have tests with names she couldn't even pronounce. Nervous and bored were bad enough, but even worse, there was nothing good to read.

She began to scour her neighbor's recycling, weekly, and brought in a fresh new stock of magazines: for the oncology waiting room, the radiation waiting room and all of the rest of the "poke, prod and deliver-dreaded-news" waiting rooms.

She also went to garage sales regularly to find toys and books for the children's oncology unit. "How awful it must be to be a child and have cancer, and be subjected to chemotherapy," she thought. Sometimes she even visited the chemo room with toys and hand puppets, to distract the children and their parents, as the poison dripped into their veins.

In a few months, Kate will celebrate her five-year anniversary of remission. Her oncologist will be taking her off tamoxifen. "Hallelujah! Finally out of menopause."

"I'm five years cancer-free. I know that doesn't mean I'm home-free. Many survivors waste a lot of time worrying about recurrences and don't do much about getting on with their lives. I figure if a recurrence is going to happen in five years, it's going to happen in five years, whether I spend my time sitting around worrying or trying to live my life to the fullest. Sounds like kind of a no-brainer to me."

Does she ever worry about a recurrence? "Of course. I have no illusions about being home-free from cancer. How could I? I'm reminded every morning when I get out of the shower and look in the bathroom mirror. But I don't dwell on it. I've got a life to get on with and that's far more important to me."

For now, the anniversary is approaching and celebration will be the order of the day. She and Paul, with a bottle of Dom Perignon, his Viagra, her falsies and their box of toys, will be off for another romantic getaway in Mexico.

"Life is good," Kate sighed. "Very, very good."

VI

PUTTING ME FIRST

MIRIAM

I'M LEARNING TO LIVE WITH CANCER

"It was graduation day. I could have called it off. The parents would have understood. But the kids wouldn't have. So there I was up on the stage in the middle of the group of kids. First, we sang "Feelin' Groovy," which was fine. Then we sang "Fly Away." I felt this powerful wave of sadness rush over me. I had to excuse myself, and let my staff finish the ceremony without me.

"I went out to my car, sat down in it, and cried. For the kids, life was just beginning. For me it was ending. The day before graduation I had gotten the results of my CAT scan. The cancer had recurred. This time it was metastatic."

Miriam had been diagnosed with breast cancer five years earlier, a year after her mother had lost her own battle with the disease. Miriam feels strongly that the stress of traveling back and forth between the coasts, only to see her mother becoming more debilitated and defeated by cancer with each visit, contributed to her developing the disease.

Miriam is Ashkenazi Jew, an ethnic group that is at high risk for both breast and ovarian cancer. When her doctor discovered the malignant tumor she moved on the disease aggressively.

Miriam was scheduled for a lumpectomy, when a small (2 mm) tumor that had showed up on her mammogram was proven by a needle biopsy to be malignant. In surgery her doctor found a larger tumor and suspected more might be discovered. Afterwards, she highly recommended that Miriam have a mastectomy, assuring her that reconstruction could be done at the same time.

Although no lymph node involvement was found, given her ethnicity, her oncologist strongly advised Miriam to have six rounds of chemotherapy just to be on the safe side.

Miriam's recovery from surgery and chemotherapy grounded her. She was unable to get out of bed for days on end, abruptly altering her lifestyle. Always an "on the go" woman, Miriam is the founder and director of a school for children with special needs, and director of a household with two teenagers and a husband who travels frequently.

"I turned over the reins for running Sunshine School to my staff. They would do a perfectly good job in my absence. I didn't have to be there on a day-to-day basis to see things being done differently than I would have done them. All I heard about was the finished product, which always turned out fine.

"Home was more challenging. I'd lie on the couch, powerless, watching my husband, Jeff, and my daughters, Sara and Judy, negotiating the running of the household. I don't know how many times I heard them arguing about whose turn it was to clean the bathroom. I just wanted to scream, 'I'll do it!' to put the discord to rest. But I couldn't."

In the recovery, Miriam found solace in quilting. She'd loved sewing since childhood. Knowing that she'd be having a mastectomy, Miriam asked her friends to bring her scraps of fabric. To her, the scraps represented her body, torn apart by surgery. In quilting, she would reconstruct the pieces to form something new and beautiful. Out of her experience with cancer, a new passion was born.

Other than her love of quilting, Miriam left the experience of cancer, and what she could have learned from it, behind. On her recovery, she jumped back into her old life at full speed.

Five years later, she found a lump on her collarbone. "Sara was home, recovering from mono. I just figured that I must have caught it from her. The fact that Sara was sick and I wasn't just slipped past me. It was only after she got better and went back to school, and I still had the lump, that I called the doctor."

Miriam called the oncologist, just to rule out a recurrence. He prescribed antibiotics. If the lump was caused by an infection, the antibiotics would take care of it within ten days. If the lump was still there, he'd schedule a CAT scan. Ten days later the lump was still there. The CAT scan revealed lymph and liver metastases.

"I was completely distraught. I was so sure that I was done with cancer. Now it was back, and it was going to kill me. Six years ago it took my mother. Last year my sister, Myra, was diagnosed. She suffered through a mastectomy and chemo, just like me. For what? Cancer was going to kill both of us, just like it did Mom."

Miriam's family wasn't much help. Miriam reasoned that everyone was so busy trying to take care of their own feelings about the recurrence that they had little left to give. Jeff loved Miriam, but he wasn't an emotional, nurturing man. The first time around, he had radically altered his work schedule to be at home most of the time. He kept the household running, took Miriam to all of her appointments, offered a shoulder to cry on, but little more. Miriam expected about the same this time.

When she was originally diagnosed five years ago, Sara and Judy were 12 and 10. Both daughters were devastated, terrified that their mother was going to die. Judy was especially affected. She missed a lot of school the first six months, feigning illness. She was afraid that if she left the house she might find her mother dead on her return.

This time both daughters were teenagers. They were as, or more, overwhelmed by their mother's illness this time, but they responded in ways that teenagers use to defend against their feelings. Sara spent a lot of time away from home. Judy stayed in her room on the phone or emailing friends.

Miriam's oncologist was gently supportive with her, always asking how she was doing and really listening to her. But he took an aggressive stance against the cancer. "We're going after it with the big guns this time," he told her. In the throes of "killer chemo," Miriam felt like it was killing her along with the disease, and wondered who would win out.

Her cancer markers were dropping dramatically. The doctor said that they had cancer on the run. He ordered another CAT scan, expecting to see nothing but improvement. What he saw were new liver metastases. He tried to console Miriam, explaining that at this point metastatic cancer is being viewed as a long-term chronic illness. There are times when the cancer suddenly appears much worse, then just as suddenly, it recedes.

Miriam couldn't hear him. "Fear consumed me. I knew that I was dying and no one could convince me otherwise. There was no plea bargaining for more time. Death was coming soon, too soon." Miriam sunk into a deep depression, refusing to see her therapist or be evaluated for antidepressants.

Just about the same time, Miriam got an email from her friend Seth, who lived in an old "hippie town" out on the coast. Seth was always getting involved in the latest New Age practice: healing, spirituality, whatever. Miriam had always considered Seth a flake, well-meaning, but no less a flake.

Several months earlier, Seth had scheduled a healing with a Tuka shaman from Russia. Knowing that she needed it more than he, Seth offered the healing to Miriam.

"I'm very anti-New Age. But Seth kept saying this wasn't New Age. This woman was a traditional healer from our ancestral home-land. 'Yeah, right,' I thought. Even if this was legit, I'm in the throes of 'killer chemo.' How the hell am I suppose to tolerate an hour's drive on a one-lane, snaky road to get there. I don't know how, but Seth won me over."

The next Sunday, two days after her latest chemo treatment, a friend drove Miriam to see the healer. "She had to stop three or four times for 'puke breaks,' but we made it."

The shaman asked Miriam very little. "Through a Russian translator, she asked my birthday and why I sought healing. Then she became very quiet. She started burning sage until the room smelled like a fireplace was backed up. Then she started chanting and beating on an animal-skin drum. The chanting got louder and more frenetic.

"At first I closed my eyes and tried to go with it, hoping I wouldn't pass out from the smoky air. But the skeptic in me couldn't stand it. I had to sneak a peek, catch the charlatan. I opened my eyes and watched her. Her eyes were shut tight and her face was painfully contorted. She was really in a trance. So I shut my eyes and let myself go with it."

After the ritual, the shaman took Miriam's hands in her own, and looked into Miriam's eyes without wavering. "Her hands were warm and reassuring. But her stare was eerie. It was like someone not human — no, superhuman — was looking through me, straight to my soul."

She told Miriam, through the translator, that she was a strong woman and she could survive this. But first, she had to overcome her negative emotions.

As she left, Miriam felt like she was in a bit of a trance herself, like her body was here but she was somewhere else. She barely spoke to her friend as they drove home. When she got home she went straight to bed and slept for twelve hours.

"When I awoke the next morning, the sun was pouring through the windows all around me, settling on the bed. It was just an ordinary thing, but it seemed so beautiful, like the clouds had cleared and the sun was shining on my life again.

"I felt weak and achy, but nothing like the way I usually feel three days after chemo. More importantly, the fear was gone. I felt strangely optimistic. I thought about what the doctor had said about metastatic cancer being a long-term illness — long-term, not terminal. I thought, 'I've got a long-term illness. What now?'

"It stopped being so important trying to figure out how long I had left to live, and I started thinking about what I wanted to do with whatever time I had left. I knew I'd never go back to work full-time. I'd given my heart and soul to Sunshine School. It was my baby, just like Sara and Judy were my babies. But none of them were babies anymore. My girls would be grown soon, and it was time to pass the baton for running the school. My staff could certainly run it. I could stay on as a consultant.

"We have property in the country. Jeff and I have said we'd move there when we retired, as if either of us workaholics could even spell "retire." Cancer retired me. I want to spend as much of the time as I have left in the peace and solitude of nature, maybe turn my quilting into a little cottage industry. Judy will go to college in three years and I plan to be at the country house full-time. Until then, I've done my fair share of the work. Jeff and the girls can pick up the slack now. If they don't do it as well as I would, it's okay."

JILLIAN

I'VE GOT A STORY TO TELL

"I found a lump in my left breast while I was in the shower. I immediately made an appointment with my primary care doctor. She examined me and found the lump. She said that there was no cause for concern. It was probably a cyst. They're common in women my age. Common in women my age? I'm 52. She told me to come back in six months."

Over those six months, the lump was Jillian's constant companion. She felt it daily, as if to reassure herself that it was still there, much in the same way that a tongue always goes to an aching tooth. It remained the same size, so she tried to convince herself that everything was okay.

After six months the doctor checked it again. She had said that if it were a cyst it would have disappeared, so it was probably a calcification; still no cause for concern.

"I know in retrospect," Jillian said, "that I should have done something, requested a needle biopsy, got a second opinion, something. But I so wanted it to be nothing that I colluded with my doctor's denial.

"I went back six months later. Now the lump was larger. I requested — no, demanded — a needle biopsy.

"I was as terrified as I was furious. I suppose I had a good malpractice case, but all I could think about was that I could die and I had to do something. As for the doctor, I never spoke to her again."

Jillian was referred to a surgeon. By the time he examined her, he likened the cancer to a horse that had broken out of the corral and was running wild.

"I told him how long ago I'd found the lump and that my primary care doctor made me wait. He asked me to tell him the whole story. He put his face in his hands and shook his head. He said how sorry he was, and that nothing like that would happen from that point on. And nothing did."

Jillian had a mastectomy and embarked on a six-month course of chemotherapy. It never occurred to her that chemo would force her to adjust and reprioritize her life. Jillian is a dynamo of a woman, with a flare for the dramatic. An ample woman with flaming red hair, and clothes almost as colorful, Jillian is unstoppable, a card-carrying over-achiever. Along with teaching first grade and being active in local politics, she was taking care of her 85-year-old father, who had Alzheimer's. She had hired a woman to care for him while she was working, and her husband, Burt, helped out, but the brunt of his care still fell on Jillian's shoulders.

After her first chemo treatment, Jillian had to hire a full-time caretaker for her father, something they could by no means afford to do for very long.

By the time she'd had her second round of chemo, Jillian was no longer able to work. The school district doesn't pay short-term disability, so they retired her. That way she could receive benefits and keep her health insurance.

At this point, Jillian was quite depressed. Her oncologist prescribed antidepressants and strongly suggested that she attend a support group. She tried a couple of groups but they didn't work for her. In some, the members were so whiny over so little, Jillian wanted to shake them. In other groups there were women who were seriously ill, and this was too depressing for Jillian to handle.

One day Jillian was talking to Juanita, the oncology social worker. Juanita said that she knew of a group she thought would be perfect for Jillian. She gave Jillian the address, day and time, but said no more.

"I laughed when I looked at the address, 120 Evans. Evans Street hadn't been the wrong side of the tracks when I was growing up. It was a working-class, primarily Irish neighborhood. There was a lot of drinking and brawling, but it was basically a safe place."

Over time, the neighborhood had deteriorated. It was home mainly to minorities, especially African-Americans. There were gang wars and lots of drugs. Still, it was the old neighborhood. Jillian's curiosity was piqued. She had to check this group out.

The group met in the basement of the Calvary African Baptist Church. Jillian entered the meeting room and was immediately aware, as was everyone else, that she was the only white woman there.

The leader, Dolores, introduced herself. The group members introduced themselves and told their stories. Jillian found one young woman's story particularly touching.

"I'm a breast cancer survivor. Actually, I'm a survivor of a lot a things," said Paulette, the small, sturdy black woman with copious braided hair and huge brown eyes. "I was diagnosed with breast cancer when I was 28. I'd just given birth to Little Eddy, my fifth child. Doctors told me I couldn't breast-feed and had to have my breast removed.

"My life had been pretty rough. My father molested me when I was nine. By the time I was 12, I was into drugs and having sex with guys to get drugs. By 16, I was an addict and a hooker. I had four children and lost custody of all of 'em. In my last bust I was mandated into rehab.

"I made it through rehab and started going to NA. That's where I met Big Eddy, my common-law husband. I stayed clean and sober until I got diagnosed with cancer. I was gonna lose a breast and I figured Big Eddy would leave. Men always left when things got rough. I couldn't take it. I started usin' again.

"Big Eddy said he loved me breasts or no breasts, and wasn't goin' anywhere. He said I had to get clean again and survive for Little Eddy. So I faced up to it. I got clean and started fightin' cancer. Cancer was the first thing in my life I ever faced up to and didn't run away."

Jillian told the group her story. She added that if Paulette could survive all she'd been through and not run away, she figured that she could do it too.

As the meeting was about to end, Dolores turned to Jillian and said, "I think I speak for the group when I say that we like your energy and we'd like you to join our group."

Jillian accepted. She knew that she was home. What she didn't know was the invaluable role these women would play in her life. She would learn the true blessing of a support group.

As expected, Jillian and Burt weren't able to afford full-time help to care for her father. At this point, Jillian could barely care for herself. Her group came to the rescue, taking turns caring for Jillian's father, helping out around the house with shopping, cooking and cleaning.

After the fifth chemo treatment, Jillian's father died unexpectedly. Under ordinary circumstances, Jillian, the strong one, the overachiever, would have organized the funeral, an elaborate wake, and made arrangements to have his body shipped back to Alabama for burial. But these were anything but ordinary times.

"I'd taken care of him while he was alive. By the time he died, I was confined to a wheelchair. For the first time in my life, I put me first. We had a small service and I had his body cremated. Burt and the girls from my group did most of the work. Mildred and Flora are gospel singers with beautiful voices. They sang 'This Little Light of Mine' at the service. It was very special."

Six months after finishing chemo, Jillian had regained her health and was ready to go back to work. The school district rehired her and was willing to let her work part-time.

"It wasn't the same. First-graders are so needy and the work just isn't satisfying anymore. My life changed so much. Having cancer brought me full circle: Dad dying and being called back to the old neighborhood to meet some of the most special women I've ever known. My life has gotten too big for the classroom. I've really got a story to tell."

Jillian wants to try writing. She and Burt don't have much money, so quitting her job is out of the question. So while she's working part-time she started taking writing classes, which she is thoroughly enjoying. On the encouragement of one of her teachers, she is starting to write her memoir. "*When a Horse Breaks Out of the Corral* sounds like a fitting title, but we'll have to see," Jillian laughs.

VII

FINDING GOD

DEBBIE

IT WAS ONLY A WAKE-UP CALL

"I was 40 and living the life of a suburban housewife. I was married to an insurance salesman. We had two small children, a ranch-style house from the fifties and a Volvo station wagon. I wouldn't say that I was depressed, but I knew that something was missing.

"My days were endless: cooking, cleaning, and chauffeuring the kids, afternoons at the mall, evenings in front of the television. My husband never questioned our life, our distribution of labor, and made it very clear that I had a problem if I questioned it. So I suffered in silence."

One day Debbie and her daughters were at the playground. While the girls played in the sandbox, Debbie sat on the bench, chatting with one of the other moms.

"I must have let it slip that I was less than overjoyed about my life, because the other mom told me that I should see an astrologer she knew. When I told her that I didn't believe in all that psychic stuff, she told me that Rob wasn't like that. He was a down-to-earth, regular guy. His charts were calculated mathematically so they had to be right. Most importantly, every woman she knew who'd gone to see him raved about how accurately he'd pegged her."

Debbie was still skeptical, but she figured that an hour or two having her chart done would break up the afternoon monotony of playgrounds and malls.

Rob's office was on the other side of town, in a converted warehouse that he shared with psychotherapists, bodyworkers and psychics. This fascinated Debbie, who had never seen anything like this in suburbia.

Rob himself looked like your basic blue-collar workman: tall, lanky, with disheveled blond hair, a warm smile and a firm handshake. There was nothing the least bit "airy-fairy, New Age" about this guy, which immediately put Debbie at ease.

She told him that she'd come at the suggestion of a friend — that she'd just turned 40 and needed some direction in her life. "I was afraid that Rob had x-ray vision and was seeing right through me — seeing that I was here because I was a confused mess, like my husband always told me I was."

Rob was quiet for the longest time as he looked at Debbie's chart. When he finally spoke, he said it looked like she'd come from a traditional, maybe Midwestern family. She appeared to be one of many children and often felt over-ignored by her parents, overlooked in favor of her more outspoken siblings. He said that Debbie had learned to put the needs of others first and become a caretaker, in the hopes of winning her parents' approval.

When she finally gave up trying to get their attention and left home, she rejected her family's values and the church she'd been brought up in. She came west seeking a more progressive, liberated way of life. Unfortunately, her old self-effacing, caretaking ways were still a part of her repertoire. She would seek out people who needed to be taken care of, but who didn't appreciate what she did for them. She would end up feeling as invisible and misunderstood as she had in childhood. Like she had as a young girl, she would try harder to be helpful and make herself needed. When she was unable to elicit the desired response, she felt like a dismal failure.

Debbie was flabbergasted. Rob's take on her was excruciatingly accurate. She wondered first how he knew all of that. Secondly, having been revealed, what was she going to do about it?

It was about the same time that Debbie had her first mammogram. Debbie rarely went to the doctor or paid much attention to her health at all. Another "playground mom" was aghast that Debbie had turned 40 and not even thought about getting a mammogram. Since the astrologer was a good tip, Debbie figured that you could learn a lot of useful things at playgrounds. Getting a mammogram probably was a good idea, so she made an appointment.

The mammogram showed a good-sized mass (2 cm). A needle biopsy verified that the tumor was malignant.

Debbie was in shock. It never once occurred to her that she was doing this because she might have cancer. She told her husband, Hal, which made matters worse. Hal had lost his mother to breast cancer when he was a boy and he equated breast cancer with death. He was terrified. Giving Debbie a grisly account of his mother's demise quickly filled Debbie with terror, too.

Debbie had been estranged from the church that she was raised in, as Rob had suspected. At this point she pretty much considered herself an agnostic. But feeling as terrified as she did, she felt like she had no other choice. She prayed. "God, please don't let me die, I have two small children. I have to be here for them."

Because her tumor was large, the doctor recommended she have a mastectomy. Debbie wasn't sure. She polled almost everyone she knew and came up with a hung jury. Since Rob seemed to know her well, without really knowing her at all, she decided to let him break the tie. Rob looked at Debbie's chart and told her to have a lumpectomy. "Cancer was just a wake-up call," he said.

In her surgery, the doctor found lymph node involvement, so chemotherapy would be required. Debbie endured four rounds of chemotherapy.

Through much of the chemo she was bedridden, in no way able to keep up with a three-year-old and five-year-old. A "playground mom" came to the rescue. She recommended a babysitter that she was quite fond of.

Mabel, the babysitter, was a large, motherly, African-American woman with a gold-tooth smile that she gave freely. Debbie's children loved Mabel.

Mabel was a devout Baptist. She talked to the girls about God, Christ and church. One Sunday when Debbie was feeling especially ill and Hal was away at a convention, Mabel took the girls to Sunday service. They loved it.

"My kids kept bugging me about church. I let them go with Mabel a few more times, when Hal was away. He didn't approve of church. I don't think he approved of Mabel either. But I was with the kids on this one. I loved her, too."

While Debbie was going through chemo she prayed a lot, asking God for guidance. Having read somewhere that prayer is asking the question and meditation is how one hears the answer, she bought a book on meditation and tried to teach herself.

When chemo was done and Debbie had regained her health, she tried but couldn't go back to the world of playgrounds, shopping malls and television. Cancer had left a gaping hole in her, a spiritual hunger crying to be fulfilled.

"My kids were still bugging me about church. They liked Mabel's, but they wanted one of their own. At the same time, I had this longing in me for something more. Rob had called my cancer a wake-up call. I clearly woke up to something, but I wasn't sure what it was."

Rob also taught meditation. He ran a meditation group that met weekly. Joining the group seemed like a logical first move for Debbie. She eagerly joined, in spite of Hal's protest.

Meanwhile, Debbie and her daughters started checking out churches. The Episcopal church felt too stuffy. It reminded her of the church she'd grown up in. The Unitarian church was a much better fit, but it still wasn't quite it. Debbie kept going to her meditation group and searching for a church.

Debbie talked about her search in her group. She was looking for a place that had what she called "traditional spiritual values," nothing New Age or cultish. But she also wanted to find a church that fostered a more direct connection with God through meditation.

One of the group members told Debbie that her church sounded like a good match and invited Debbie to accompany her the following Sunday.

From the outside the building looked like any other. There was no steeple or cross indicating that it was a church. But the parishioners were dressed in their Sunday best: men in suits and women in flowery spring dresses. The children were clean-scrubbed and on their best behavior.

Inside the church had rows of chairs, flowers and candles, like any other church. But the altar was quite different. There was a picture of Jesus and a statue of Mary. Along with them were more exotic pictures and statues that seemed to have a Middle and Far Eastern flavor.

In the ceremony there was singing, chanting and meditation. The ministers spoke not only of Holy Father, but also Divine Mother. There was something called a purification ritual. Each parishioner, if he or she chose to, could write on a piece of paper a quality in themselves that they wanted to change. Then they would approach the altar and cast the paper into a fiery caldron. A minister would gently touch him or her on the hand and pronounce them purified of the trait.

By the time the two-hour service had ended, Debbie knew she had found what she was looking for. She remembers looking at her friend from the meditation group and whispering, "This is it, I'm home."

Over the next two years, Debbie and her daughters became active in the church. She found the sense of community she'd been looking for, first in "playground moms," then in Rob's meditation group.

In the meantime, Debbie and Hal drifted further apart. Debbie was no longer the subservient, self-effacing woman that Hal married. She had found a deeper meaning in her own life and was no longer interested in "piggybacking" his. She suspected that Hal, who had moved further away from the relationship himself, was having an affair. It was never confirmed. Over time their marriage dissolved.

Years later, Hal confessed to Debbie that it began with the cancer. He was so afraid that she was going to die that he willed himself to stop loving her, so that he could buffer himself to what he saw as an inevitable loss. In a sense, he was right. He didn't lose Debbie to cancer. He lost her to finding herself.

Coincidentally, when Debbie's divorce was becoming final, she started hearing about a residential community that her church operated. She visited and took the community tour. She knew that she'd come home.

Debbie has been a resident and active member of the community for fourteen years. She raised her two daughters, who've gone away to college. She found herself and her place in the world. Cancer was just a wake-up call, and has never recurred. But Debbie hasn't forgotten or failed to remain grateful.

"Without cancer I may never have found God or home."

JULIE

FINDING THE PATH OF MINDFULNESS

"I'll never forget the day I got my diagnosis," Julie said. "It was January 28, 2002. I was 45. My mother was diagnosed at 45. She was dead by 50.

"I went home feeling completely shell-shocked. All I wanted was for Mark, the man I'd lived with for six years, to hold me and tell me everything would be okay. But Mark had news of his own. He'd fallen in love with someone else and wanted to be with her. I was devastated.

"In the course of twenty-four hours my entire world had been shattered. I didn't think that I'd ever be able to put it back together again. I didn't even know if I wanted to."

Julie wanted to have her surgery yesterday. It was as if extricating the intruder from her body would break the evil spell, render the whole thing simply a bad dream. She'd wake, Mark would hold her, let her cry and reassure her. Then she'd count her blessings, thankful that it was just a dream.

Unfortunately, or fortunately, Julie's surgeon couldn't operate on her until the end of February. Julie couldn't simply have the situation surgically removed. She had to live with it.

Julie is a tall, willowy brunette. A university professor by profession, her soft-spoken directness barely hints at the well of strength within her — strength she would need to survive the next year of her life.

"Thank goodness I'd been taking a class in mindfulness meditation. When I couldn't just escape the situation, I decided to try to be present with it, moment to moment. It was excruciating at times. But I almost made a game of staying present, no matter how bad it got," Julie remembers.

"I spent the month between my diagnosis and my surgery mourning my own death. I journaled about my life: the joys, the sorrows, what I'd learned, what I'd lost, what I was never to experience. Despite all the pain, it was strangely comforting.

"When I went into surgery I was serene and peaceful, almost joyful. Nobody had any idea what to make of it, including me."

Mark felt terribly guilty about having committed the heinous crime of bad timing. He stayed with Julie through the early course of treatment and took her to all of her appointments. Two weeks after surgery, she moved out.

She had a pretty easy time with her surgery, which she credited to her great attitude. Because she had a large (3.5 cm), aggressive tumor, with four lymph nodes involved, chemotherapy would be required.

"I reasoned that since my great attitude had served me well in surgery, it would continue to work its magic in chemo. Boy, was I ever wrong."

Mark was planning to take Julie to her first chemo treatment. He called twenty minutes before her appointment. He was tied up in a meeting; she'd have to get there on her own. He'd pick her up afterward.

"It was at that moment that I realized that this was what our whole relationship had been like. I had wasted six years of my life on a man who was only interested in himself, his job, being seen in the right places, driving the right car. I was the one he'd come home to. I'd comfort him, support him, take care of him, and kid myself that I was getting something in return. I had asked almost nothing of him during those six years. When I finally did, he couldn't come through."

Julie pulled herself together and walked to the hospital, arriving ten minutes late. "I sat in the chemo room alone. I've never felt so alone in all my life. I tried to be present, observe without judgment or attachment. I wasn't doing very well with it, but at least it helped pass the time."

Mark showed up, fifteen minutes before the treatment ended, and drove Julie home. She was already feeling the effects of the toxins and threw up all over his BMW. "A fitting farewell," she thought.

Julie had four chemotherapy treatments, each one more debilitating than the one before. She would have a treatment every three weeks, then spend the next ten days in bed.

"I'd taken a two-semester, unpaid leave of absence from the university, and I didn't have much money. I ended up taking this dumpy little apartment that was next door to a sleazy bar. It was noisy: music, people yelling, fights breaking out, all hours of the day and night. There I was in bed, feeling like hell, being subjected to it. The landlord took pity on me and let me out of my lease. Between chemo treatments two and three, I moved again."

When chemo finally ended, Julie was cast adrift. As hellish as the whole thing had been, it had given her something to focus on, something to summon her courage to get through. When it was over she felt like there was nothing left. She had mourned her death, and in a sense, she had died. So, who was left?

She decided to take a road trip back to the childhood she'd long left behind. She needed to know where she'd come from, who she'd been, who died.

Julie remembered very little about her early childhood. She was born in Iowa. But the family had lived in so many places in the Midwest that she never really knew where home had been.

Her father worked as a disc jockey and changed jobs frequently. In reality, he had a hard time holding down a job. He'd lose a job and her mother would keep the family afloat, taking in sewing, cleaning houses or waiting tables. Eventually, her father would either find a job or the family would reach the point where they could no longer come up with rent money. Either way, it was time to move; usually abruptly, sometimes in the dead of night.

"I have one vivid memory. I was five, and had just started kindergarten. I was making friends and finally feeling like I belonged somewhere. We needed to get out of town, fast, probably for the usual reason. My parents packed the car on Sunday night. We were on our way out of town before dawn on Monday. We passed my school as we left town. I cried and cried, knowing that I'd never be going back there," Julie recalls.

Her parents divorced when Julie was a teenager. She hadn't seen or spoken to her father in over thirty years. She'd escaped home into an ill-fated marriage at 18. She occasionally spoke with her mother, but never saw her in person until she returned home, at 27, to be with her when she died.

With a map, a list of towns, a few street addresses, and a name or two of people who might remember her family, Julie set out for the Midwest.

She drove from town to town. Sometimes, she found a school that looked familiar, or a park she thought she might have played in. Occasionally, she found a house she thought she might have lived in.

In Salina, Kansas, she met a former neighbor who remembered her family. "Mrs. Williams remembered that a couple of times a year my grandmother would send my sister and I frilly pinafore dresses. On Sundays my mother would dress us up for church. She took great pride in sending us out in clean, starched and ironed dresses, and carefully polished Mary Janes. I hadn't remembered any of this."

Julie didn't really learn much about her family on the trip. At first she felt disappointed, that the trip had been a waste of time. Eventually though, the mere act of making her pilgrimage seemed to suffice. She was satisfied that she knew where she'd come from well enough to finalize closure on the first half of her life. The girl she'd been in the first half had died, and made way for the woman she would be in the second half, to be born.

"I'm really looking forward to the second half of my life," Julie said. "Through cancer, I've learned that life is precious and sacred. I want to live as fully and consciously as I can, each and every day.

"I have no illusions about the future. I had a large, aggressive tumor, with lymph node involvement. I know I'm not done with cancer. I don't really expect to live more than ten more years.

"I know it sounds morbid and depressing, but I don't feel that way at all. I feel like cancer has given me a second chance. I feel like I've been able to free myself of a lot of the falseness in the way that I'd been living my life, so that I can live more authentically.

"I see a lot of women who had breast cancer, living in fear of recurrences. Some put their lives on hold for a year, or two, or five. They won't eat anything that isn't organic or ever have a glass of wine. They just exist, waiting for some kind of sign to tell them they're home-free, and can start living their lives.

"Not me. I see each day as a gift, and living it as fully as possible as an act of gratitude. Recurrences are going to happen regardless. Why not just live in the only time you know you've got — today."

Julie continues her mindfulness meditation practice on a daily basis. It has led her to an interest in other Buddhist spiritual practices. Periodically, she goes on weekend and longer meditation retreats.

On one of these retreats she met Erik. Like Julie, Erik had suffered tragedy and loss, and grown from the experience. Three years ago a drunk driver killed his five-year-old daughter, and only child. A year later, his marriage fell apart, unable to hold up under the strain the tragedy had put on it.

Julie and Erik felt a strong, immediate sense of connection. Neither one was looking to meet someone, or felt ready to get involved again. Still, one thing led to another, and their relationship quickly grew and deepened.

"The ordeal of going through cancer made me grow up. And I'm finally capable of having an adult relationship. My relationship with Mark was really pretty adolescent. I tried to be who he needed me to be, tried to make myself indispensable to him, so he'd never leave me. It backfired. Now I feel like I have a strong sense of self that I wouldn't abandon for the sake of a relationship. I'm really ready to meet someone like Erik."

Julie was very honest with Erik about the breast cancer — that she expects it to recur and doesn't expect to live long enough to grow old with someone.

Erik's response was, "Many people run from pain and suffering, and end up living lives that amount to little more than existence. Only by opening yourself up to life, with all its pain, can you open to life with all of its joy. And that's the only life worth living. I'd rather have ten years with Julie, or five, or one, than a lifetime without her."

He proposed. She accepted.

VIII

THE HOLY WOMEN

IRINA

SURRENDER

Irina was only 15 when her mother died. But she remembers it vividly thirty years later, as if it happened last year.

"My mother protected her husband and children from her illness. By the time we knew, her cancer had metastasized and she was very ill.

"Unlike most Russian women her age, my mother was literate. She loved to read. She read to us when we were little. Sometimes, she even read to us when we were older. As the cancer in her brain grew, her sight diminished. Finally, she went completely blind.

"My mother also loved to sing — old Jewish songs she'd learned as a child. She had a beautiful voice. When the cancer invaded her lungs, the tumors took over. She could no longer breathe deeply enough to sing. Medicine in Russia was very primitive compared to America. They couldn't even provide her with an oxygen tank to help her breathe. In the end, I think she just suffocated."

That was Irina's introduction to breast cancer: a sort of demonic force that takes over a woman's body and smothers it to death. For years afterwards, she would wake screaming from nightmares. The cancer armies had been invading her body, again.

None of the family handled her mother's death well. Her father seemed to simply withdraw from life and died himself, two years later. Although the medical cause of death was vague, Irina, to this day, swears he died from a broken heart.

A year later, an 18-year-old Irina and her sisters, Tatiana, 21, and Alexandra, 24, immigrated to the United States. Their mother had a cousin in Los Angeles. They'd never met her, but they'd found her address in their mother's papers. On the chance that they could locate their only relative in America, they packed up everything they owned and bought one-way tickets to Los Angeles.

The sisters found their relative, who helped them settle in. Tatiana found a place for herself and stayed. Irina and Alexandra were still searching for something: something to explain and give meaning to what, up until then, appeared to be a cruel, meaningless world. They were both drawn to the teachings of the late Indian guru, Paramhansa Yogananda. Two years later they moved to the Sierra Nevada mountains to live in a community of his followers.

Initially a monastic community, it had become a householder community, where members married and raised families. Both sisters met and married young men in the community, though neither had children.

In 1999, Alexandra, then 45, started missing her periods. She noticed the waistlines of her slacks and skirts getting tighter, and she was experiencing nausea and strange abdominal pains. She and her husband, Matthew, had prayed so long for a child. Alexandra thought that at last God had answered their prayers.

When the results of the pregnancy test came back negative, Alexandra didn't understand why the doctors wanted to run more tests. She was given a sonogram and then, with a fine needle, the doctor extracted brown fluid from her abdomen. Finally, the doctor apologetically delivered the results. She had stage VI ovarian cancer.

Because the prognosis was so poor, Alexandra agreed to have a total hysterectomy, but declined chemotherapy. She chose to spend the last months of her life peacefully, with her husband, her sister and her community.

"The last two weeks of my sister's life were spent in the county hospital in town. The townspeople are apprehensive about us. They think that we're weird, religious fanatics. Some even call us a cult. I think the people at the hospital, anyway, got the opportunity to see us more clearly.

"Alexandra's room was like a shrine. Community members were there all the time. People were meditating or praying silently, or chanting softly. It was so peaceful, it changed the whole mood of the hospital. I think everyone felt it.

"Master teaches us that we are not the body. The body dies, but the spirit is eternal. So death is not a cause for sorrow, but for celebration, since our spirits have been freed of the earthly body. Unfortunately, most people did not grow up believing this, and no matter how devout their spiritual practice, they have a lot of trouble surrendering their hold on the earthly body.

"A few days before her death, Alexandra was lying in her hospital bed, barely strong enough to speak. She was holding Matthew's hand with one hand and mine with the other. She whispered, 'This is the hardest thing I've ever done.'

"Something changed over the next few days. She floated in and out of consciousness. When she opened her eyes for the last time, she looked at me, with a beautiful, serene smile, and whispered, 'Celebrate.'"

Being an Ashkenazi Jew, Irina is at high risk for ovarian and breast cancer. When Alexandra was diagnosed, the surgeon suggested Irina have a prophylactic hysterectomy. Irina had no problem with this. "I'd already decided against having children. And I've never equated my femininity or my identity as a woman, with my plumbing. Having a preventative hysterectomy made sense to me."

Shortly after Alexandra's death, Irina had her first mammogram. There was a shadow on the film. The doctor wasn't particularly concerned, and just asked her to have another in six months.

Irina, on the other hand, was very concerned. Because of her ethnicity she asked to be tested for the BRCA gene. Her test came back positive.

"I was hysterical. I knelt in front of the altar and prayed, 'Master, just get me through this thing and I'll have my breasts cut off.' I asked the surgeon for a prophylactic mastectomy. He refused. The same man, who wanted to get rid of my ovaries and uterus wanted to preserve my breasts. For what? For my husband's sake? He was on my side."

Six months had passed and Irina had another mammogram. This time, things went quite differently.

"The technician took the usual pictures and went into the other room to look at them. She came back and told me that she needed more pictures, took them and left again to look at them. This time she was gone a long time and I was really starting to worry.

"When she finally came back, she told me that I needed to go down the hall for a needle biopsy; but she wouldn't say any more.

"A doctor performed the biopsy and I waited for another eternity. Finally, he came back and said that he was sorry, but that I had breast cancer. He was sorry. I wasn't. All I could think was that now I can finally have this thing taken care of, once and for all. And that's exactly what I did. I had a bilateral mastectomy."

Although the doctor found no lymph node involvement, he strongly recommended chemotherapy because of her family history.

"The surgery was no big deal," Irina remembers. "But the chemo was a nightmare. I've always been an active person. I'm director of the community's business services office. My husband and I enjoy running and hiking. After chemo, I was so exhausted for days on end, I couldn't even get out of bed and make a cup of coffee.

"I got quite depressed. My husband was wonderful, but, I'm sure that I was pretty hard to be around. I kept trying to do something, when all I could do was nothing. One day I was lying in bed, nauseous and exhausted, and I looked up at the wall, at my guru's picture. I knew, in an instant, what I had to do: surrender — totally, completely surrender.

"People have always thought of me as a courageous person, coming to this country as a young girl, not even knowing the language. But my life has always been ruled by fear. I have always been terrified of being abandoned. My mother abandoned me, then my father, then my sister. I was afraid of cancer taking my life or the lives of the ones that I love. I tried hard to control my life: stay healthy, be a good wife so my husband wouldn't leave, be a good devotee so God wouldn't abandon me. In that moment I realized that I had to surrender that fear. I had no choice.

"It took cancer to finally make me surrender. Surgery is the mutilation that brings humility. But only chemo is strong enough to annihilate the ego and bring surrender.

"Since cancer I'm a happier person, a less fearful person. I'm a better person. I'm a better boss, less controlling, more compassionate. I'm a better wife, more loving and trusting. I'm a better devotee, because I've learned to surrender my will to God. But, I've learned that it's not a one-shot deal. I have to keep practicing compassion, trust and surrender, every day.

"I don't know what the future holds. Who would know? I hope for a long, healthy life. But my life is in God's hands. I can live with that."

TERESA

DIVINE UNION

The late-afternoon sun filtered through the frayed lace curtain covering the window of the small wood cabin. The light comes to rest on a frail woman in a rocking chair, snuggled in an afghan in spite of the warmth of the August afternoon. Her cane rests close to the chair. Sparse tufts of newly sprouted gray hair cover her head. Her lined, chiseled face, suggesting wisdom, is complimented by her soft brown eyes. Her presence feels ethereal, almost holy.

Teresa speaks softly. "I was drying off after my shower when I found the lump under my arm. I was startled. It seemed quite large and I thought it had probably been there for quite awhile. My heart sank, because I knew that it was serious. How had I not noticed it before?

"I hadn't seen a doctor for a long time. I rarely go into town. And I don't believe in allopathic medicine. I usually just rely on herbs. The truth is that I fear I'd kind of forgotten my body. It's a pitfall of the spiritual path. My church believes in healthy living and natural healing. But, when you reach the point that you're meditating for several hours a day, you start to forget your body. Then you get a rude awakening like this that says, 'I'm still a being in a body.'

"I made an appointment with the clinic in town. My suppositions were confirmed. It was very serious. It was breast cancer, stage III or IV, the doctor suspected. I would need to go to the county hospital for more tests.

"The doctor there recommended a mastectomy and four rounds of chemotherapy. I went along with the recommendations, not because I necessarily agreed, but because it would buy me some time to decide what I wanted to do.

"The doctor kept emphasizing the seriousness. He never exactly said that I was dying. I guess he couldn't manage something like that. He did say that I would probably need to repeat the chemotherapy more than once," Teresa remembers. "I thought, 'We'll see.'

"The hospital sent me to see the breast cancer nurse. She gave me all of this information and referred me to web sites. I guess this is what most women want, information, so that they can feel less powerless with their disease. I wasn't interested. I guess I'm not as afraid of feeling powerless. I don't know. The nurse ended up being pretty annoyed with me."

Teresa went through her surgery and initial chemotherapy treatment almost unconsciously. A perplexed friend from her church commented, "It's as if Teresa's body is going through treatment, but she's somewhere else. I wonder if this is what a lifetime of meditation does for you. If so, I'd better practice harder."

Then one morning, shortly after her first chemo treatment, Teresa woke in excruciating pain. "I've never experienced pain like this. I'd get a stabbing, burning pain in my back. Then, it would shoot down my left leg. I'd clutch myself in a ball and the muscles would go into spasm. As soon as one round was over, another would begin.

"I crawled to the phone and called my neighbors. They got me into a chair. I couldn't lie down and I couldn't really sit up, so they kind of propped me up in this chair. They called the doctor and got me some pain medication. Someone had to stay with me twenty-four hours a day, to help me get to the bathroom and to feed me. It went on like this for three days.

"Ordinarily, I'm pretty much of a loner. I live alone, don't really socialize. It was hard to ask for help, even though my neighbors are members of my church. I was overwhelmed by the love and care people showed to me, especially since they hardly knew me."

After three days Teresa was comfortable enough to be driven to the hospital for tests. An ultrasound revealed a mass between her third and fourth lumbar vertebrae. A CAT scan proved it to be malignant.

"Now, I was scared, really scared, and confused. I kept thinking that this can't be happening. This is the worst thing that's ever happened to me. Then, a very soft voice said, 'This is the best thing that's ever happened to you.' Then I knew what to listen to, and I calmed down.

"I had radiation every day, as well as chemotherapy every three weeks. In my first radiation treatment I was lying on the table when the strangest feeling came over me. I felt like I was safely in a womb. It's very hard to explain. But I knew that God was holding me, keeping me safe. The radiation was rays of divine light. And I felt so much better after just one treatment."

What Teresa realized she had experienced was a moment of oneness with God. Yogis call it *samadhi*, divine union. She had glimpsed it in meditation, but never anything like this.

"It brought me great joy and peace. I'd try to get back there, when I was in the throes of chemo-induced illness. But like the old adage says, you can't petition the Lord with prayer.

"Occasionally, I could return to that blissful state. But most times I just had to be where I was. I'd read Saint Teresa of Avila. She spent her whole life in so much pain and still did such great things. Feeling like a wimp in comparison made me feel better.

"A lifetime of spiritual practice and meditation prepares you for the experience of oneness with God. That I'd known for a long time. Cancer taught me why this is so. The ultimate experience of oneness with God comes with death.

"It's said that when Gandhi was shot he called, 'Ram, Ram, Ram' — the name of the Lord. He had spent his whole life preparing for death. When it came, he was ready.

"Death gets bad press in this culture. It's as if people say, 'I don't want to die now because I'm enjoying my life so much.' The truth is that they're suffering a lot. If they can put death off for awhile they can buy themselves some time. Then maybe they can figure out how to stop suffering and start enjoying. Then, of course, they wouldn't be ready to die, because they would be enjoying life too much. In this scheme of things, death is never convenient," she laughs.

"It's not like I'm preparing to die tomorrow. At the hospital, they say that my cancer numbers are down, whatever that means. They kid me and say I'm like Lance Armstrong. I came in on my last legs and walked out healthy.

"It doesn't matter when I do die. Cancer has vividly reminded me that I will. For this, I'm grateful. So, if I slip up a little — think a drive up the coast or a movie would be nice today, better than meditation — I'm reminded. I see the doctor every two months. If that's not enough, I just look over there." She looks towards her cane.

"I have permanent nerve damage in my leg. I can't walk without a cane. But it's good, because it reminds me.

"I'm having a little sciatic pain in my right leg now. It's probably nothing. I'll mention it to the doctor when I see him next month, if I remember."

She smiles. Darkness blankets the room.

JOY

FAREWELL PARTY

"I remember the first time I saw her. It was the Memorial Day picnic and she was playing volleyball with some kids. She was slight and fair, but deceptively strong. Her long auburn hair was tied back. And her eyes, I can still see those laughing hazel eyes.

"What could I do? I jumped into the game. She welcomed me with a smile. We laughed and played, while kids were beating the pants off us.

"She was the most joyful, luminous soul I've ever known. Her parents weren't spiritual people. They must have unconsciously been channeling something when they named her Joy."

Dave met Joy the year after each of their first marriages had ended. Actually, they had known each other, though not very well, years earlier. Joy's college roommate became Dave's first wife. Occasionally, Joy would pick up the phone when Dave called and they would chat briefly, or they'd see each other at a party.

When Dave married, he and his wife left Portland and the spiritual community where they all lived. He spent the next ten years on the East Coast. When his marriage ended, the East had come to feel like alien territory. He quit his job, packed up his meager belongings into his VW bus and headed home, to Portland. He arrived two weeks before Memorial Day.

Dave and Joy were inseparable that summer. They found that they had so much in common. Along with being long-time members of the same spiritual community, they both enjoyed living simply, loved animals and the outdoors. They never seemed to run out of things to say or do together.

"I kept thinking that it was too soon. Both of us were barely out of our first marriages. But, I knew. I knew that Joy was the woman I wanted to share my life with. She felt the same way about me."

In October, Dave and Joy were married amongst the loving well-wishers of their community. They embarked on what they both expected to be a long and happy life together.

The next spring, Joy found a lump in her right breast. She had lost her left breast to cancer five years earlier. She's had a mastectomy and one chemotherapy treatment. That was all it took for Joy to conclude, "I'm just not a chemo kind of gal." Fortunately, she went into remission anyway.

Now, she was 44, the same age that her mother had been when she died of breast cancer. Joy was happier than she'd ever been in her life. She was married to a man that she loved dearly, had great friends and a loving community. She feared that the cancer had recurred, threatening it all.

She made a doctor's appointment. The doctor wasn't worried. Thinking that it was probably a cyst, he elected to take a wait-and-see attitude. He told Joy that if it was still there, she should come back in six months. Given her history, this was a terrible mistake.

"In retrospect, I know I should have done something: made sure that Joy got a second opinion, had a needle biopsy, something. But she came home so relieved. The doctor had given her tacit permission to go into denial. I went right with her. We were so happy that we just climbed into a magical bubble that projected us from the harsh reality of the situation… for awhile longer, at least."

The lump didn't disappear. Joy returned to the doctor six months later. The bubble was irrevocably burst. The tumor had grown. It was malignant, aggressively invading fourteen lymph nodes. (When ten or more nodes are involved, the prognosis is poor.)

Joy underwent a radical mastectomy, removing the breast and all of her lymph nodes. Doctors talked about aggressive follow-up treatments: six rounds of chemotherapy so strong that Joy would have to stay in the hospital while having them; then a bone marrow transplant in which her entire immune system would be destroyed and she would spend months in hermetically sealed isolation. No one spoke of these extreme measures as curative, only as a way of extending her life a little longer. Without further treatment, they gave her one year to live.

"Joy and I were both numb. She had no intention of subjecting herself to such brutal procedures. Our friends kept trying to reassure us. These were just numbers. We should stay optimistic, have faith. She's gone into remission before without all of the excesses of allopathic medicine. She could do it again. We were now, I fear, experiencing group denial.

"We didn't do anything special that year, since we weren't buying into this year to live hokum. We served God, lived our lives, loved each other, until time ran out."

It was spring again. One of the fiercest winters they'd seen in years had finally yielded. Now, new life was peeking out everywhere. Spring was Joy's favorite time of year. She delighted in seeing the new buds burst open, finding a bird's nest full of tiny blue eggs, and seeing the wobbly fawns with their mothers dining in the garden.

In April, Joy's chest grew red and swollen. Her chest, shoulder and arm felt stiff, and she kept trying to stretch out the stiffness. She went to see the doctor who confirmed that it was the cancer.

Within a week or so, her lungs filled with fluid. She could no longer lie down. She slept sitting up at the dining room table, her head propped up on pillows. Finally, the swelling became so uncomfortable that she went into the hospital, where they drained her lungs.

"Joy went into the hospital in mid-April. I kept on working, stopping by the hospital after work. Then a friend who'd lost his wife to breast cancer a few years before confronted me. 'Look, man, she's dying. What are you doing?' My denial was finally broken. From then on I spent every waking and a number of sleeping hours at the hospital with Joy."

On May 1, Joy went into crisis. This time her heart sac, not her lungs, filled. Draining it was much trickier. Joy was in the ICU and the doctors were draining her heart sac when she stopped breathing. The hospital alert for code blue sounded. Doctors and nurses rushed into the ICU. Dave and Joy's brother, Rick, rushed in with them.

"Rick and I started chanting 'Om,' which is what you do when someone is dying. Joy started breathing again and regained consciousness. 'Chant Om Divine Mother,' she commanded. So, we chanted Om Divine Mother. She told us to chant the names of various saints. Then she told us to chant Om Arjuna. We looked at each other puzzled, then did as we were told."

"Joy had this very close friend whose spiritual name is Arjuna. He was there for her through her divorce. They were like brother and sister. That morning, Arjuna was working in the store in town when he had this overwhelming feeling that he should come to the hospital. About half an hour after we'd chanted his name, he walked into the ICU."

After a day in the ICU, Joy's condition was considered stable. She was moved to a room on the third floor — the "dying floor."

Her denial finally broken, Joy went into action and got ready to die magnificently.

Firstly, she got on the phone and called everyone with whom she'd had conflict to make amends. "She called her ex, which went well. She called my ex, which didn't go so well. But Joy was not to be dissuaded. She cleared the air from her side. People would ask me if she should be doing all of that. After all, she was dying. I felt that she knew what she was doing. She was dying her way."

Next, Joy called friends from the community. "I'm dying. Please come to my farewell party." Within a few hours her room was full, with people spilling into the hall.

For the next three days, loving friends came and went; food and flowers came in a steady stream. People slept in the hallway. The hospital didn't interfere. Joy had won them over too.

Joy laughed and joked through it all. "Give me a kick. Maybe I need a push, or a pull, from the other side. Maybe they don't want me on the other side. What if this is a big joke and I'm not going to die.

Dave will take me home and I'll get hit by a truck on the way."

The second day Joy was still in high spirits. Her friend John, the astrologer, called. "How are you?" he asked. "I'm trying to die," she answered. "I think you read my chart upside down."

Joy blessed each person who came to bid her farewell. They shared a few moments, remembering some endearing or funny anecdote from the friendship, hugged their goodbyes.

Someone asked Joy if she was leaving anything unfinished. "No," she answered. "There are a million things I'd like to do. But I've had a full and joyful life. I have no regrets."

Joy's spirit was strong, but her body kept getting weaker. She took morphine every four hours for pain. Her face was so thin and her eyes looked so big, just like a child, radiating this wonderful spiritual energy. "Joy looks like Divine Mother," one friend commented. "Oh, go on," responded Joy, throwing a box of Kleenex at her.

But a divine energy did permeate Joy's room, and poured out into the rest of the hospital. The bastion of cold, mechanistic, allopathic medicine was, unbeknownst to itself, transformed by her presence. Doctors and nurses would stop by with flowers when they were going off shift. They would say goodbye; it was an honor to have served her.

On the evening of day three, Joy's pulse weakened and her breathing became more intermittent. She drifted between waking and sleeping.

"By 4 a.m., the room was quiet. Joy was withdrawing from us. We whispered words of encouragement to her, to go into the light. I tried to hold her hand. She pulled it back and she was lost to me.

"At 5 a.m. her breathing became very quiet. She took ten to fifteen more breaths. Then she was still. She wasn't mine anymore. She wasn't ours anymore. She was with God."

EPILOGUE

In Buddhism it is said that we wake up, but then go back to sleep. The same could be said about breast cancer. After her initial diagnosis a woman's knee-jerk reaction is typically, "I'm going to die." Since most women diagnosed with breast cancer will have non-invasive cancer (DCIS) or moderately invasive cancer, their treatment will likely be a lumpectomy plus radiation; a round of chemotherapy only if there is lymph node involvement. They will complete treatment, their lives getting back to normal, the "I'm going to die" will fade into the background and breast cancer will remain only a vague memory. It is unfortunate that so few take advantage of their "mortality wake-up call" as an opportunity to examine their lives and grow.

I spent a year and a half interviewing women and one man (who lost his wife to breast cancer) who didn't go back to sleep. When the furor of the "I'm going to die" passed, it was replaced by a quiet, more inquisitive "I'm going to die?" These women were contemplating their own mortality. Since breast cancer is a trickster, it only offers remission not a cure, these women had no way of knowing whether the rest of their lives would mean fifty more years or only five. They didn't have time to waste. They asked the big questions: "Who am I? What's important to me? What do I want to do with my life?" Then, they took action.

A Woman's Initiation was birthed within my own life. In 2002 my best friend was told that breast cancer had recurred. This time it was metastatic. She struggled, and I struggled with her to find meaning in this cruel, senseless disease. On July 3, 2004, quietly, with grace and dignity, Patricia gave up her struggle. I struggle on. I give voice and money to search for the cure. More importantly, I champion the cause of using a breast cancer diagnosis as a springboard for finding a greater sense of self, and creating a more authentic, satisfying life.

Diana Murphy
December 14, 2004

THE AUTHOR

Diana Murphy is a licensed psychotherapist with eighteen years of clinical experience. She works in private practice in San Francisco, where her clients are primarily breast cancer survivors.

The author received a master's degree in clinical psychology from Antioch University. She lives in Mill Valley, California, and divides her time between her four great loves: writing, practicing psychotherapy, long-distance running and mountaineering.